Praise for *Write Yourself Home*

"The first step to telling the truth—in your life, on the page—is letting yourself *hear* the truth. Johanna's practice of embodied writing offers a way to access the truth that lives in the body, beneath other ways of knowing. You won't find a wiser, more compassionate teacher."

—MEGAN DEVINE, best-selling author of *It's OK That You're Not OK*

"For anyone whose body has rewritten their life without permission, *Write Yourself Home* offers a different way forward. Grounded in somatic awareness and radical permission, this book offers accessible practices for those navigating illness, trauma, grief, or burnout—without pushing, fixing, or bypassing. Designed to be done from bed, from rest, from wherever you are, Franzel helps readers reclaim their own language, agency, and sense of wholeness—without denying pain or demanding recovery. This is not writing to improve yourself, but writing to come home to yourself. Highly recommend."

—SARAH RAMEY, musician and author of The Lady's Handbook for Her Mysterious Illness

"This spectacular and deeply resonant book shows us an entirely new way to pay attention to our bodies. *Write Yourself Home* is an enthralling, luminous, deeply moving account of a descent into illness and a path back to the body and to allegiance to that body, through language. In her deeply innovative and beautifully curated exercises, Johanna Franzel shows us a way to open up again to life and to hope and joy and full embodiment. Find a cozy chair, because you won't be able to put this book down."

—SUSAN CONLEY, author of *Landslide*

"An essential guide for every body. *Write Yourself Home* invites you to fully inhabit the life that's yours, and it does so with creativity, warmth, and clear steps. I highly recommend this book to every single person out there who happens to have a body!"

—STEPHEN COPE, author of The Great Work of Your Life

"In *Write Yourself Home,* Johanna Franzel reframes the basic act of writing. This is a writing process that pays a different kind of attention and provokes new form and meaning from the knowledge you carry around with you everywhere. What is truly revelatory is watching Franzel demonstrate, through her own experience, how to use writing to follow the instructions of the body. Then she shows you how! This book is deeply generous, practical, and accessible. You will walk away knowing just what to do."

—CHANA JOFFE-WALT, radio journalist and producer at *This American Life*

Write Yourself Home

Write Yourself Home

A Creative Guide for Living Well in the Body You Have Through Embodied Writing and Movement Practice

Johanna Franzel

North Atlantic Books
Huichin, unceded Ohlone land
Berkeley, California

North Atlantic Books
Huichin, unceded Ohlone land
2526 Martin Luther King Jr Way
Berkeley, CA 94704 USA
www.northatlanticbooks.com

Cover design by Jess Morphew
Book design by Happenstance Type-O-Rama

Printed in the United States of America

Write Yourself Home: A Creative Guide for Living Well in the Body You Have Through Embodied Writing and Movement Practice is sponsored and published by North Atlantic Books, an educational nonprofit that collaborates with partners to develop cross-cultural perspectives; nurture holistic views of art, science, the humanities, and healing; and seed personal and global transformation by publishing work on the relationship of body, spirit, and nature.

North Atlantic Books's publications are distributed to the US trade and internationally by Penguin Random House Publisher Services. For further information, visit our website at www.northatlanticbooks.com.

The authorized representative in the EU for product safety and compliance is Eucomply OÜ, Pärnu mnt 139b-14, 11317 Tallinn, Estonia, hello@eucompliancepartner.com, +33757690241.

CONTENT DISCLAIMER: This book contains material that may be triggering, including references to self-harm or trauma.

Cataloging-in-Publication Data available from the Library of Congress
ISBN
Print: 9798889843627
Ebook: 9798889843634

1 2 3 4 5 6 7 8 9 KPC 31 30 29 28 27 26

For Jon and Nora

You may do this, I tell you, it is permitted.
Begin again the story of your life.

—Jane Hirshfield, "Da Capo"

CONTENTS

PART IV NAMING. GRIEVING. CELEBRATING.

PART V DISCOVERY

PART VI CONNECTION. COLLECTIVE. SONG.

AUTHOR'S NOTE

In 2003, I walked out of one of my first meetings with a gastroenterologist holding a thin pamphlet the doctor had given me. It featured an illustration of a neat, winding digestive tract drawn in hues of pastel, under the title *Your GI Tract*. Surrounding this image was the nearly transparent outline of a young, white, trim, apparently able-bodied man. I knew the picture didn't represent me or my ailing GI tract, but it clearly communicated what the medical system regarded as a "normal" or "standard" body.

Dear reader, as we embark on this embodied writing practice, let's tear up the pamphlets and dispel any assumptions about what constitutes a body. Let's do away with the notion that someone else can represent your body. Instead, as you move through these practices, please embrace your own precise shapes, expressions, and histories. Offer yourself radical gentleness and abundant permission to amend what's offered here to fit your own capacities and curiosities.

While my own experience is with a digestive disease, we won't be privileging any particular illness, loss, body part, or experience. Some of the material you'll find here is sensitive and medical in nature; please take your time or step away as needed. This is a work of narrative nonfiction based on my own experiences as a patient, practitioner, and human. I've done my best to reconstruct dates, scenes, and conversations, and have changed most names throughout. *Write Yourself Home* is meant to accompany you as you come to inhabit your own body, but it is not a substitute for the additional support you may need. And what you need matters. I'm so glad you're here.

INTRODUCTION

My body did not break all at once. It broke so slowly, in fact, that for a while I could pretend everything was fine. Perhaps our opening scene, the one in which I finally begin to grasp the reality of what's happening, is this one: It's the spring of 2007, and I am curled up on the bathroom floor, wedged between tub, sink, and toilet, tears streaming down my cheeks. I should not be here. In fact, at this very moment, I'm supposed to be 200 miles away, setting off on a multiday charity bike ride for sufferers of inflammatory bowel disease. Sure, I shared this same diagnosis, but I was capable and resilient, helping those who were *truly* sick. Which again, wasn't me. But now my symptoms rage so flagrantly and undeniably that I cannot get up from the floor or pretend that what is happening *isn't* happening.

What is happening: electric pain that makes me keen. A face so swollen from prednisone it looks ready to sail off my body. I told people I was having "belly problems," but the truth was further south and less quaint, in an ulcerated colon that would not stop its endless flaring. Blood and mucous exited my body at all hours, which meant that any place that wasn't a bathroom was a calculated risk; I was constantly discovering new levels of humiliation as my insides spilled, grossly. Inflammatory bowel disease is a chronic condition in which the immune system attacks the entire digestive system. The inflammation didn't end at my colon but extended throughout my body: swelling on my skin, sores in my mouth, rashes that flamed across my limbs, hands, and once, inelegantly, onto my eye.

There on the floor I could no longer deny the burning, exhaustion, and pain that racked my body or perform the trick that made my ambitions louder than my condition. I knew I wouldn't be getting on a bike that day, I wouldn't be following through on my heroic fundraising efforts, and I wouldn't even be leaving the bathroom. Instead, I'd have to confront the terrible truth: How I felt might actually matter more than the competence I was trying to prove.

But let us stay in this scene a bit longer, and we'll see that I am reaching for something blue and spiral bound. Because there is a place where my body speaks honestly of its conflagrations, and it is there, tucked beside me. A notebook.

When I finally stop crying, I open this little journal, pick up my pen, and turn to the first blank page. If we are really paying attention here, we might notice the tiniest shift; my breath slows and softens. There is a small feeling of relief that whatever impossible feeling I'm holding has somewhere to go. And then I write. I write my humiliation and heartbreak. I write from the crackling directness of my body's experience. I write because I don't know what else to do. I write because the story I've been telling about myself is just beginning to come undone, and writing feels like the only way through.

Looking back on this scene I feel such compassion for this scared, isolated version of myself. I wish I could whisper to her that even if her symptoms wax and wane—which they very much will—she has taken the first step toward something that will carry her through all of this with abiding generosity: She has allowed the truth of her body to inform her words. This seemingly small move will deliver her, and eventually many others, into a very different kind of life. One that doesn't turn on how well she performs capacity but makes abundant space for the truth of her condition, opening the way for discovery, connection, creativity, and joy. Decades on, I'm still astonished by the radical repair that's possible when we engage the creative process in our bodies. Maybe you've felt this too: Connecting to your body's knowing through writing is a pathway to your own vitality and larger health.

Words have always mattered to me. I wrote through teenage angst, heartbreak, falling in love, new motherhood. I taught writing to middle schoolers, helped teenagers write their own radio stories, and crafted essays and audio pieces. So as my life came undone, the only thing I knew to do was write. Only this time, I was moving directly from the urgency of my breath and sensation to the page, and it was . . . different. Back in the early aughts, I'd never heard the word *embodiment*. I had no language for what I'd later recognize as somatic work, which guides the antennae of our awareness inward to the subtle, mysterious sensations pinging beneath consciousness. But I knew this: The more I wrote this way, the more I understood that my writing and my body were in a vital conversation, one taking place beneath my canceled plans and disappointments.

And there were so many. A few years later, when I was hospitalized for nearly a week, I wandered the halls like a lost skinny ghost, an IV pole in one hand and a notebook in the other. When my hands broke out in blistering pustules, effectively ending my new career as a massage therapist, I found comfort in writing. Projects that were interrupted, careers and relationships that had to end—at every turn, writing from my body helped me find solace and vitality amid the mess. Writing was a place where my body, in all its complexity—its aliveness as well as its suffering, its nuance and knowledge—could express itself on the page.

This was not the story being told in my ever-growing medical file, which flattened my experience into a lifeless series of numbers and scales. The medical system was certainly keeping me not-dead, but it seemed to have no way of recognizing the parts of me that were alive. For that, I needed language that seized back the truth of my own experiences, and my writing had been doing just that, linking me to my body's knowing, my own knowing. The more I paid attention, the more I encountered my body as a friend, one with clear boundaries and an audible *no, thank you* (and sometimes, as when a doctor suggested a sigmoidoscopy without anesthesia, *no way*). This didn't lead to the cessation of my symptoms or suffering, but something more enduring: a willingness to show up as my whole self and regard my life as something that mattered.

As a teacher, I knew this bodied kind of writing was a practice that needed to be shared. What I didn't realize was that my trajectory—which kept circling education, storytelling, and the body—was helping me assemble precisely the training and experience that I needed to share it. I earned a master's in education focused on storytelling and the arts. A training in documentary writing and radio honed my ear for voice and storytelling. As my health disintegrated, interest (and desperation!) led me to a degree in neuromuscular massage that offered tactile learning in anatomy, health, and tissue structures, and eventually to biodynamic craniosacral therapy, which refined my understanding of the nervous system, presence, and subtle body movement.

My experience includes decades teaching, working in public radio, and practicing somatic bodywork with clients both on the table and in online embodiment sessions. Underlying all of this was the deep schooling of my body, breaking insistently over twenty years, calling me back again and again to mystery, to bearing honest witness from within, to my own voice—on the page and out loud. Along the way, I was guided by many teachers, colleagues, clients, and students who showed me what transformation through embodiment looks like and that their healing was not separate from my own.

In 2015, I decided to try the wild experiment of turning my studies, my somatic practice, and my experience with writing into a workshop I offered at a friend's studio. The idea was simple: We'd combine gentle breath and body exercises with writing prompts and optional sharing in something I called *embodied writing*. I tacked up small flyers around town with the invitation, "Come see what happens when you invite your whole self into the room." I held my breath—would this even work?

But from that first session, it was clear: Embodied writing was transformative. Over the next ten years, the work bloomed into hundreds of workshops, online gatherings, work at cancer centers, refugee organizations, and community programs for disabled artists. In each space, I watched people move into their bodies and then connect, in writing, to a voice that was distinctly their own. The ingredients were so simple, but magic was happening in those rooms. People fell in love with their writing, with each other's words, with their distinct, authentic selves.

Most of us need guidance and instruction on what listening to our bodies means. We need specific questions that invite exploration and permission to move, write, or be quiet in our responses. Folks who take my workshops never fit into a single category, but they do come with willingness, they come with a hunger for spaces that invite their whole selves, they come trusting that anything infused with permission and reverence will have space for them. Even if we can't control our symptoms or our sensitivities, we can listen in a way that connects us to the ripeness of our intuition. Connects us to potency. Reclaims writing as a site of authenticity where we touch what's true and life-giving and possible. Where we name, remember, and create.

In these pages, I'll share the gentle somatic practices and writing prompts that transformed my life—and eventually the lives of many others—so that you too can learn to inhabit your body with more trust and healing, regardless of histories or symptoms. *Write Yourself Home* isn't a how-to on creative practice so much as a guide to an accessible and life-affirming form of expression, one designed to support any reader, regardless of background or experience, to reconnect with themselves and their bodies.

Most of us don't practice connecting to our bodies, and we have good reasons not to. Because of illness or trauma, loss or anxiety, hearing the cues of our body can feel both impossible and dangerous. Add to this the modern experience of a life mediated through our phones and, oh, the fact that we're rewarded for paying more attention to outside expectations than interior feelings, and you begin to understand why embodiment can feel so off the menu of regular life, why disconnection might seem like the sounder, safer option.

If you've found your way here, you might be feeling the chafe of this estrangement. Perhaps you're getting through your days but not feeling really present or quietly withstanding a lengthening list of discomforts. Perhaps you suspect that there's more to this ride than the treadmill of work or self-improvement. Maybe, like me, you're trying to manage a chronic illness that's thoroughly disrupted your life.

You don't need to identify as a writer or as someone with illness or trauma to receive the benefits of an embodied writing practice, which are abundant: fortified self-trust, deeper fidelity to your own felt sense, and language to name what's true. But also, life *feels better* from here. Looser, easier, and more supple. Embodied writing can help wake us up to our lives, deepening a sense of presence and play. Whatever has brought you here, to this page and this moment, my hope is that the writing and embodiment tools in this book, developed and honed over years of teaching and practice, allow you to reinhabit yourself with a greater sense of knowing, care, and even joy, reclaiming your own fullness and permission to feel it all.

If we measure a body by how it succeeds or fails, we can miss the whole dang thing. We turn a complex ecosystem into a two-dimensional line. What a too-small frame for something that is creating the miracle of being alive every damn minute. But more dangerously, when we flatten ourselves this way, we might come to believe the myth that we are failing at life or are somehow outside life altogether. Which, speaking personally, is a rather seductive story when you are bed bound and fragile. Friends, we're here to dispense with that lie altogether. I promise you your life isn't elsewhere. Even if social media tells you otherwise, even if you haven't left the house in months.

Your life is here, it's in you, and you can feel it and write it and practice exercising the muscles—creative and figurative—that situate your life in the center of you. In these pages, I'll offer you practices that help you inhabit yourself from the inside. Embodied writing turns to the life that's right here, even bedridden, even overwhelmed. I'm hoping we can build a space where you encounter your words in surprise and revelation because they come from some loosened-up place inside, some bodied place that isn't performing an okayness you don't feel.

Words matter. *Your* words matter. Language that only describes us from the outside can do real and lasting harm. Not only medical language, which can flatten our experience, but dominant language that marks us as too little or too much or unworthy or any category we aren't defining for ourselves. My own experiences have made me a fierce advocate for the importance of claiming our own language from within. When we do, we develop an inward relationship imbued with care, creativity, and presence. Writing becomes an act of love. Writing into that love helped me recognize, with surprise and delight, the vitality that had been there all along.

I've designed the practices and guidance here to accompany you on your own explorations from the comfort of your own house, and even your own bed, if need be. We'll follow the arc of one of our workshops, moving from grounding and settling to naming, discovering, and connecting.

Our chapters will be brief, digestible, and deceptively simple. They are baby steps in the truest sense: small, radical discoveries that seed an entirely different way of moving through life. You'll find abundant practices and tools, short essays for guidance and story, evocative scenes from sessions and workshops, and first-person reflections on embodied writing in action. The appendix includes instructions for practicing with a group, and you can find links to audio meditations on my website, johannafranzel.com.

Because my life and work are nourished by a vast web of teachers, you'll find inspiration drawn from poets, dreamers, scientists, practitioners, and clients. I extend deep gratitude to them, and also to the lineages and bodies upon which all of this knowledge rests. That includes earth body, seasons, tides, animals, and wisdom that is spoken, sung, prayed, and planted with a grace not necessarily codified in written words.

All of our embodied writing workshops begin with this acknowledgment: You have a body. Your own remarkable body with its particular histories, desires, experiences, expressions, and wisdom. Let this be a space where you are guided by what calls to and compels your own singular body. Here we are incubating something important, and it is not the ability to follow directions or look to a barometer outside of ourselves. Let your body, *yours*, be your guide. May these tools help you align with the possible, the mysterious, and the bodied. May they support you in reconnecting to what you've always been: beautifully, utterly alive.

PART I

Orientation

Welcome, acknowledgments, container-setting, getting resourced.

Embodied writing begins with this truth: You have a body. Here at the beginning, we incubate a space guided by the body and its knowing, slowing down to inhabit ourselves more fully and explore resource. As we reconnect, we lay the groundwork for understanding practice and orient to foundations of embodied writing.

WHAT IS EMBODIED WRITING?

At its core, embodied writing is a simple practice: A gentle physical exercise (breath, movement, stretching) followed by a prompt, and writing. If we're writing in a group, we might share our words aloud and reflect back to each other the parts and passages that moved us. Simple. *And yet.* There is a freshness to writing from the only place you actually are. When I get into my body, I find rooms I haven't opened in decades. A light comes through the cracks of my old stories, revealing an entire ecosystem of memory, sensation, and presence. I am not alone in this discovery.

Not long after I offered my first embodied writing class, I started noticing that different varieties of this approach to creativity existed in many different spaces. It was almost as if some invisible mycelial network of writing and body awareness had infused the field, and we all seemed to be responding to a call to tune into our bodies and explore the stories we carry. Psychiatrist Bessel Van Der Kolk's seminal *The Body Keeps the Score* certainly planted seeds, bringing ideas around trauma-sensitive care and somatics to the mainstream, but other scholars and writers have preceded and followed his work. Psychologist Stephen Porges and clinician Deb Dana's research and teaching in polyvagal theory offer new perspectives on the socially connected aspects of the nervous system and treatment tools for dysregulation. Writer and embodiment teacher Prentis Hemphill, writer and pleasure activist adrienne maree brown, and author and activist Sonya Renee Taylor have all been leading voices in anchoring a somatics dialogue rooted in collective care, anti-racism, and justice.

Against this backdrop, no wonder embodied writing was springing up all over the world. Psychologists, dancers, trauma therapists, writing instructors, yoga teachers, in works like Laraine Herring's *Writing Begins with the Breath* and Lisa

Weinert's *Narrative Healing*. Perhaps we didn't share a singular lineage, but we all were compelled by the potent alchemy of embodiment and writing. For me, embodied writing emerged out of necessity—my own breaking body demanded more authentic expression—but it was also a return to something I'd almost forgotten.

It took me years to discover—or, more accurately, *remember*—that writing could be playful and loose. Because in the beginning, language was joy, and I let it rip. I was the kid who told long, rambling adventure stories, wrote epics of time travel and fantasy, and sang loud. When we would visit my family in Sweden, I spoke the language freely, unencumbered by my own large gaps of grammar and vocabulary.

And then, with a thunk, high school. I lost something when words became *Words*—rarefied, careful, judged—and the life was snuffed out of them. Where once my voice was boisterous, it became wispy and questioning. I "learned" a good deal, but a kind of deliberateness crept in, a dull stiffness I took as the *right way to do it*.

So many of us know this experience; once our writing gets held up to the harsh light of graded standards it becomes leaden with conformity. Suddenly, our wild, creative stories are not *good* writing. As a teacher, I can appreciate the desire to give students a shared set of tools. But from the student side, writing became synonymous with judgment. No wonder so many of us shrink at the prospect of being called *a writer*, as though this mantle requires a special kind of earning. This is one reason I dreamed up embodied writing workshops around the assumption that whatever emerges is perfect. We celebrate rather than critique, undoing decades of thinking that we are only writers when we conform to a regimented set of rules, have some sort of mystical talent, or know a secret writing code. All of which are lies.

My embodied writing classes were borne out of a deep longing for this freer, original connection to language, one that I had and then lost. My colon, that great teacher in humility and humiliation, finally drove away dull habits and called me back in, demanding I recover this joyful, bodied voice that was willing to follow the wild path of its own curiosity. And this is my hope for you too, that the practice lets you hear the bass note of yourself again, offering something to dance to. When we begin our practice by literally moving, we lose the stiffness and remember not to take this all too seriously. What new ideas ever came from rigidity anyway? There will be time to polish later, but here we are working with ignition, with generation, with loosening up the life inside and bringing it along.

Living with chronic illness has shown me that I forget my body at my peril. If I deplete my reserves, pushing myself into shapes and places I cannot sustain, I'm ravaged. Not visibly, but inside there is a kind of leaching. And if I keep going, pulling from the aquifer too long, too much, the consequences are dire. My margins are thinner, but they're not unique. All of us who attempt to armor over our feelings, forgetting ourselves and our bodied, mysterious knowing, enter a kind of stiff lifelessness. We cut off creative discovery, shutting down the wondrous, the intuitive, the bodily. Here as we begin our practice, we're bringing tender awareness to these old habits. We're slowing down to reconnect inwardly, laying the groundwork for a different kind of support.

So what is embodied writing, really? It's claiming our bodies as a place of knowing and language. It's opening the aperture on awe so that we might step into our own lives. It's waking up to the subtle body and building capacity for noticing how we feel—really feel—away from prescription or explanation, as a way of informing what we see and make and name. It is reclaiming your own original, bodied voice and letting it rip.

Setting the Foundations
THE SIMPLE STEPS

We're nearly ready to explore our own embodied writing practice. As we begin, it's helpful to name some simple steps that will help anchor you in the process. Pausing for a moment in these foundations allows the body to soften and the writing to bloom.

1. **Begin where you are.**

   I'm writing this on a bracing February morning in Maine, with the winter sun bright through the kitchen window, and the air still enough that if I step outside, I can just make out the sound of the ocean a mile or two away. Embodied writing starts with exactly this: acknowledging where you are. And not just where you are, but the long, peopled history of that place. The many who tended this air and water and land over generations. That still do.

   Here in Southern Maine, I'm standing on the indigenous homeland of the Wabanaki Confederacy. Locating ourselves like this nests us in time and space, deflates that old saw of the lonesome, rarefied writer. We aren't first or last. Just here. And so we begin with the particularities of here: this day, this place, this moment.

2. **Know that you have a body.**

   A body with its own needs, paces, rhythms, shapes. Your own, singular, luminous body. Let this be a space where you incubate listening to what you actually need, where you become more intimate with the language of your organism and what it wants, perhaps that's as simple as a glass of water or an extra breath.

   This is no facile instruction. Acknowledging ourselves this way widens the lens on our subtle bodies, letting us begin to pick up the quiet cues, feedback, and sensations we might otherwise plow right through. If we are going to find language for our real experience, let us practice *not* withstanding and come into our body's deeper awareness. Doing so cultivates a softness that makes way for new stories, ones that may arrive less like a bolt of lightning than a subtle emergence. "Inspiration comes very slowly and quietly," writes journalist and writing teacher Brenda Ueland. "This quiet looking and thinking is the imagination; it is letting in ideas. Willing is doing something you know already, something you have been told by somebody else."[1] When we orient to an inner compass, we might perceive the difference between willful trying and the intuitive inspirations that come with allowing.

3. **Offer abundant permission.**

   Permission says: Please follow the call of your actual you. Be wide with yourself, be inclusive. If the prompt doesn't speak to you, or you feel like napping, or if what you're actually compelled to do is eat chocolate and stare into space, then that is your actual work. Which sounds simple but is deep medicine for those of us who have spent lifetimes under the mantle of *have to* and *should*. We celebrate breaking a rule if that rule takes us away from ourselves. It's worth a pause here, dear reader, to return to yourself and see what happens when you soften your bracing, let your shoulders fall. What surprises might come from *not* trying so hard?

   The truth is that in this work we're repairing habits of schooling. We want to change what we value most from *what we're told to do* to *what we're called to*. A productive embodied writing session is one in which you are a joyful ally to your creative self.

   Of course sometimes, especially in the midst of turmoil or illness, it can feel difficult to discern what we want other than *not this*. Which is why we need permission all the more. *Not this* is enough, it is plenty. Let our practice be spacious enough to hold whatever we're carrying.

4. **Invite Reverence.**

   If permission reminds us to get wide and loose with ourselves, reverence calls us inward to the temple of our attention. Think of the way you might gaze at a newborn or a seascape. In front of this magnificence, you rarely use a corrective lens, thinking, *yeah, she's cute and all, but couldn't her eyelashes be longer? Couldn't that seagull move to the right?*

Reverence says: *Oh, my. What a wonder this is.*

Reverence invites us to bring this blueprint of awe to whatever emerges in the process, to regard ourselves and our writing with appreciation for the very miracle of existing, exactly as they are. Enough. If you find yourself drifting into self-doubt, see if you might breathe into those knotted-up places, maybe even summoning a reverence that sighs, *Oh, my. What a wonder this is.*

5 & 6. **Name how you are and what is well.**

Now let's take a moment to name and set down anything that might be distracting us from really arriving here (a recent call with health insurance, unfolded laundry) and to identify a place, movement, or moment that resources us, that feels good. "Resource" is key to this practice, and a theme we'll weave throughout. Resource orients us to what is well, nudges us to explore what good actually *feels* like. For me, resource can take many forms, depending on my energy and mood. The copper-red fur of our sweet dog Rosie. The smell of cardamom. My daughter, Nora, singing to herself in the other room. Feel free to get playful and expansive as you listen for your own resources.

7. **Know what we don't do.**

Embodied writing is not about critique. We're here to foster your emerging and generative practice. Despite what school may have taught you, please avoid poking, analyzing, or otherwise trying to improve what's already just right. Instead, build your capacities for noticing what is well by leaning into a wider kind of listening. Notice the images, words, and phrases that sing. If the language moves you, perhaps even repeat what resonated. *Dust motes in a shaft of light. Filaments of cold. I carried you in my mouth.*

8. **Speak out loud.**

Speaking your words matters. Even when you're practicing alone, try reading aloud to yourself, your pets, your plants. Moving the words from the page to the voice completes a quiet loop: beginning in the body—writing on the page—returning to the body. Not everything wants to be shared, but allow the possibility that something might, even a sentence, a word.

The ingredients are so simple, really. Basic. But it is radical to experience this kind of inclusion and witness. It is elixir for your self-knowing and your writer's voice. And it begins to whisper in ways you can actually hear that all of you gets to come along, without condition. Again and again, I've been gobsmacked by how nourishing and alive writing feels when I've moved from these foundations for practice, offering myself a genuine invitation to show up fully.

In these pages you'll find a variety of tools to help you discover embodied writing on your own. Each practice begins by setting the frame for what we'll explore, offers an invitation to engage body, breath, or imagination, and ends with a prompt to get you writing. Many practices include steps to deepen and integrate the material. All you'll need is a pen and paper, and a bit of space and time. Bonus if you have comfortable clothes, a beverage, and delicious treats nearby. Setting a timer is optional but can provide a supportive container.

And now, with our foundations laid, we can begin to move and write. My hope is that these exercises bring you closer to a sense of inhabiting yourself from within, and that as you begin to trust your body's sensations, insights, and knowing, you write—and maybe even live—in ways that include the whole of you.

Let's try this out.

Practice

BEGIN WHERE YOU ARE. TAKING (INVENT)ORY

Now that we're oriented and have our foundations, we're ready to dive into our first embodied writing practice. Grab a pen and paper, get comfortable, and let's begin.

In this first exercise, we'll practice the fine art of noticing what's right here while tuning our senses to what resources us—what delights, fortifies, or otherwise feels good—even if it's not in the room. And because finding our way to the present moment takes practice, we'll summon the *invent* part of *inventory* to ease the way in. We can catalog what's here and also let our curiosity roam, casting a wider net to listen for what's possible.

Engage the Body

Begin by settling into your body. Let your eyes soften or close and loosen your jaw and shoulders. See if you can work a little less hard to be right where you are. (For added support, visit johannafranzel.com for a five-minute audio meditation on settling and grounding.)

Then, bringing your awareness to your breath, inhale to the count of five, and then exhale to the count of five. Repeat this inhale/exhale for four rounds. As you slowly open your eyes and bring your vision back into focus, begin to take in your surroundings.

Write

Some of you may be familiar with this exercise as a tool for calming the nervous system; it can also help us move into presence while imagining possibilities.

1. Make a list of five things you can see from here.
2. List four things you can touch from here. Notice how granular you might be, how fine-tuned (*eye lashes, comforter, pen*).
3. What are three things you hear right now? If the answer is nothing—linger a bit. I've been amazed by how many sounds my younger students could find underneath supposed quiet if they kept their ears open. (The scratching of your pen and the heater hum count as sounds.)
4. List two smells you notice from right where you are.
5. What is one thing you can taste, right now (*your own saliva, the tea you just sipped . . .*)

Now pause for a moment and let your lens widen. We're going to revisit this list, but this time we're listening for what we love or enjoy.

1. What are five things you love to see but that aren't necessarily visible from here? Feel free to call in dreams and fantasy, to really be inventive. *My beating heart, a perfectly made bed, an ice pop stand under a beachfront palapa . . .*
2. What are four things you love to touch?
3. What are three sounds you really love hearing? I'm partial to spring peepers and water glugging out of a nearly full bottle.
4. What are two smells you love?
5. What is one thing you love to taste? Feel free to get carried away if this becomes a longer list.

Add to these lists at any time, letting this be a living conversation between what is here and what brings you alive.

Deepen

Is there anything that's distracting you from writing or tugging at your toe? Make a list of what you're setting aside so that you can fully arrive here.

Practice

GREETING THE BODY

Your body has been with you the whole time, through all your moments. The ankle sprain in high school. The grief at your grandmother's bedside. The flying leap you took into the lake. Regardless of how you inhabit it, your body holds memory, experience, posture (and this is only a partial list!); it holds knowledge. Connecting with that knowledge can be both a practice and a compass, a way of locating what feels true and resonant. In this exercise, we start a conversation with our bodies *in which we listen*. And because most conversations begin with a greeting, we'll do the same.

Engage the Body

Please take a moment to gently say hello to your body. Beginning from a sitting position, start by mobilizing your spine, rocking from side to side, and arching your spine forward and backward (in cat/cow for those familiar with yoga postures). Feel free to engage your head and neck.

Roll your shoulders forward and back, then lift your shoulders to your ears on an inhale and release them on an exhale. Repeat this a few times.

Gently find your way to standing and lightly bend and straighten your knees, wiggle to your toes, and roll your eyes. (You're welcome to do this from lying down as well.)

Letting your arms be heavy and your knees loose, imagine you're wearing a coat with too-long sleeves. Then, begin to gently sway side to side, allowing your arms to swing out and gently tap the opposite hip, alternating so that hands cross in front and behind your torso. Repeat five to ten times, taking care to only turn as far as feels easily comfortable. Please adapt the movement to your own body, making adjustments by slowing down your arms, only moving your eyes from side to side, or simply imagining the movement.

Finding stillness, let your attention widen to include your whole body. Start to listen from different sites. Perhaps focus on your feet, your lungs, liver, palms, ribs. Just noticing each part from here.

Write

Choose one of these sites in your body (or more, if you're drawn to more than one) and write in response to: *What my ______ (hand / colon / heart, etc.) knows.*

Deepen

As you move through your day, try listening from different sites in your body. See if you can bring curiosity into your exploration of what your body knows, maybe even offering kind words to acknowledge its insights.

Practice

EXPLORING RESOURCE / WHAT *GOOD* FEELS LIKE

When the grief of the world overwhelms, I try to hold close the words of poet Saeed Jones: "Gotta have some sweetness in this life. I believe in the intelligence of honey."[2] *The intelligence of honey.* When our seriousness gets brittle, we can sometimes forget that pleasure has its own deep wisdom.

Connecting with resource—with *what feels good*—fortifies our ability to move out of the ruts of habit. And let me say clearly, this practice isn't about bypassing or ignoring what isn't well. We're not looking for silver linings or punishing, everything-happens-for-a-reason nonsense. This is simply an invitation to loosen our grip, summon curiosity, and let our attention settle on anything that spurs pleasure, which may or may not include our physical body. Truthfully, there have been days when a glass of water was the only resource I could genuinely identify. But that was enough to bring me some sweetness.

Following are two paths for exploring your resources, one vigorous, good for shaking off cobwebs, the other slow, perfect for languid days. Whichever you choose, see if you can stay curious about what good feels like *to you.*

Engage the Body: Energetic Version

Breath of Joy is a wonderful way to shake things up. From a standing position (or seated, making sure there's room to extend your arms), take three sips of air inward, moving your arms with each inhale: first out to the front, parallel to the floor, then out to the side, also parallel to the floor, and finally up above your head. On the exhale, let the air really gush out, letting your arms descend beside you, maybe bending the whole top of your body down as you do so.

This exercise is truly vigorous! Remember to listen to your own energy stores as you gauge what exertion feels appropriate today. A single round (three sips of air inward, one exhalation) may be plenty; repeat for five to ten rounds if that feels available.

Write

Things that bring me joy . . .

This could be a list! Loud music, soft socks, birdsong—let whatever comes to mind out on the page. A five-minute time limit may help.

Engage the Body: Gentle Version

Play with moving as though honey is lubricating your joints, imagining slow, thick, fluid movements. Put on a song to sway to or try transitioning from sitting to standing in a honeyed way. Is there a piece of music that feels like the right soundtrack for inhabiting this mellifluous slowness? Nina Simone's "I Want a Little Sugar in My Bowl" certainly comes to mind. Then, letting your imagination roam free, allow your senses to guide your exploration of *good.*

Write

What good feels / tastes / smells / looks / sounds like . . .

This practice often puts me in a joyful reverie! *Good smells like popcorn. Sometimes tastes like pickles, capers, olives, brine. Good comes galloping out of a bad mood when my friend calls.*

Deepen

In Ross Gay's *Book of Delights,* he set out to write a bit each day on a moment of delight. His catalog of ordinary wonders makes room for the complexities while celebrating the particulars: a crossing guard, sunlight, garden, shoulder pat from a stranger. *What might you include in your own catalog of delights?*

Practice

PERMISSION SLIPS

Do you remember the permission slips you brought home from school? The ones a parent or guardian were supposed to sign, granting you permission to get on the bus or go to the science museum? Mine always ended up crumpled at the bottom of my backpack, and maybe I understood permission this way too: something flimsy, granted from the outside.

The first time I understood permission as freely available, it was through my friend Matthew Burgess's *Permission Slips* project. Matthew is an author, poet, and educator with an eye (and ear) for playful attention. Over several years, he used his camera to document evidence of permission, which he would pair with titles that made the connection explicit. A woman jumping into blue-green water was named *Permission to Take the Plunge.* Roller skates stowed in the corner: *Permission to Be Prepared.*

Matthew's images ignited something, as if anyone could sign off on permission: Yes to all of it. When I tried this out for myself, I got looser and more playful. Even bedbound, I found evidence. The geranium buds on the windowsill became *Permission to Break Out.* Leaves outside my window: *Permission to Fall All the Way Down.* Rather than a force granted by some outward authority, I began to sense what permission might feel like from inside.

Engage the Scene

Spend a few minutes looking around for *evidence of permission.* Once you've settled on an image, scene, or object nearby, see if you can capture this image using your camera, making a small sketch, or simply using your eyes. Beginning with *Permission to . . . ,* just write down a title that you'd give this scene. Feel free to be deeply ridiculous (and to break up the structure of the sentence)!

Engage the Body

Imagine that you could dissolve any trace of *have to* or *should* from your own body and instead soak in a sweet bath of *however you're moved to be,* moment by moment. From a seated position, see if you might bring a little sway into your spine, following the impulse toward whatever direction compels you. Could the movement begin to include your head or shoulders? Perhaps you've found yourself bouncing, slowing, quickening. Stay with this movement for a few breaths, and then begin to notice what happens if you consciously invite permission to infuse different areas of your own body, like your back, belly, face, or hands.

For me, I notice that when I invite permission into my body I feel a bit softer, looser, wider. My breath deepens; my back softens. The feeling is a little like the quiet after the vacuum finally clicks off: I didn't notice there was noise, but now that it's gone, I'm relieved. Remember that *any* response (feeling nothing or not liking this exercise at all) is just right. We're simply noticing, seeding the field of what's possible.

Write

Whatever you noticed (or didn't!), take that experience onto the page: *Permission feels like . . .* (Perhaps permission feels like sun on water, like my body after a swim, like canceled plans . . .)

Deepen

There's a peaceful stream in the woods near my house, and when I visit it I notice an inward softening that reminds me of permission. As you become more familiar with the feeling of permission, are there places where you notice this feeling is more available?

FIRST PERSON

Permission as the Truest Call

In this first reflection on embodied writing in action, writer and naturalist Bridgett Brunea shares an unlikely insight by way of fried mushrooms and a jolt of joy.

It was our second week of Johanna's online course, Writing Ourselves Awake. I had just rushed home from work, preparing dinner quickly before our Zoom call began. There wasn't time to eat before class started, so—vaguely thinking that I should focus on writing and eat after class—I placed my dinner on the stove nearby, where it was now calling to me with delicious aromas while my stomach rumbled. I was particularly excited about the fried mushrooms I'd made and kept looking at them longingly while we began introductions. Despite my hunger, a hazy, half-conscious sense of the "right way" to do this whole writing thing kept me rooted in my seat, quiet and grumpy and mushroomless.

After a few minutes of this self-inflicted hanger, Johanna gave us a writing prompt to play with: "Things that bring me joy." Something about the word *joy* jolted me awake. It was then I realized the irony of what I was doing: *denying myself food in a class about embodiment,* all because of some strange, culturally inherited notion that ignoring my bodily needs is simply the way to do things—in life and in writing.

Realizing this, it became immediately obvious what I wanted to do. As our writing time began, instead of picking up a pen, I grabbed my plate. In that moment, I gave myself permission to set aside my writing and respond to my body's actual needs. I savored my food, I began to feel better, and words started to playfully jostle around inside me. In the last few minutes of the writing period, I found myself smiling as I wrote a single line: "Things that bring me joy: eating fried mushrooms when I'm supposed to be writing."

When I read this line aloud a few minutes later, everyone laughed, myself included. It was a small victory in the direction of permission, but it felt significant, and I could feel the delight it engendered rippling through the group, as well. Not only had I respected my body—giving myself the permission and reverence on which embodied writing is formed—but through that, I had also written something that sparkled with aliveness. It didn't matter that it was a single, unprofound, intentionally silly line. It felt mischievous; it felt excited; it felt *awake*. And in writing it, I began to feel those things in myself too. Writing what I actually wanted from a place of genuine respect, gentleness, and bodily listening had cultivated something real and enlivening. It was diminutive, it was silly, but it was *alive*.

Later in the course, I was delighted to find that this little line became a touchstone of permission that others would occasionally mention with an impish grin. This didn't happen because it was a life-altering magnum opus, or because it kept my classmates up at night with its continual revelations. It happened because it was imbued with the qualities of permission and reverence that invigorate our writing and our lives. We've been culturally trained to de facto deny our actual wants and needs, even in the name of creativity. This experience made me wonder: What if, instead of following the cultural dictates of grinding productivity as I write, I could actually listen to my body and my life as I create, crafting something that feels alive and enlivens me in the process?

In some alternate reality-version of this experience, I could have labored away at a string of words that meant nothing to me while my stomach continued to rumble. I would have been hungry, produced boring writing, felt bad the whole class, and forgotten the experience entirely. Instead, I listened to my body's needs, and in the process, Johanna's beautiful tenets of permission and reverence became real to me in a way I have never forgotten.

Was my writing that night profound? Did it make me weep with recognition? Did it change the direction of my life? No—but it gave me joy, it made me laugh (such true medicine), and it reinforced a sense of my own autonomy, both in writing and in life. We get to listen to our bodies as they actually are while we live and create, and in claiming that, we become more joyful, more whole, more awake human beings.

That night, I realized a delightfully anomalous truth—that the truest call of embodied writing might not always be *writing*. The words we create are not the point. It's the energy behind them, the energy they cultivate and encourage in our lives and the lives of others, that are really what this whole writing thing is about. Even a single line—sparkling with energy and rooted in bodily joy—becomes something worthy of writing.

WHAT IF ALL IS WELL?

Sometimes life makes obvious, dramatic moves. The birth of a child, a decision to leave or stay. These are singular decisive moments that shift everything, dividing the timeline into before and after. And then sometimes, a small seed drifts in, plants itself in the foundations, and slowly begins to break up the asphalt of what you thought you knew.

Crisp mid-September 2013. A friend was hosting a visiting teacher from Colorado and asked if I wanted to go to her talk titled, mysteriously, "What If All Is Well?"

Of all the simplistic, bypassing fairy tales, I thought. I had a toddler at home, a job in public radio, a menacing disease that routinely exploded across my life. This, inside a world of supreme inequity, loss, and heartache. *What if all is well?* We were barely getting by over here. But I was interested, and so, out of equal parts curiosity and defiance, I went.

As we settled in, I noticed the teacher, Margaret, standing at the front of the room. She was dressed in soft fabrics, layers of purple and red, and radiated a steady warmth. She practiced something called biodynamic craniosacral therapy, and her voice was disarmingly gentle.

"In this practice, we help people see that there are other possibilities that are available to them; we do this by guiding our attention to what is in movement rather than what is static." She paused. "How can the story be carried differently?" I was familiar with story—years in public radio and grad school meant I often thought in stories—but I'd never really considered how stories were carried or lived within a body. I certainly never imagined the body itself as a guide for a more habitable or healthy life. But that's what the practice seemed to center. From what I could tell, biodynamic craniosacral therapy was a hands-on modality involving attunement to the subtler rhythms of the body and nervous system as a means of healing. I could not explain the technicalities, but something about Margaret's words resonated, and I felt my armored cynicism beginning to soften.

"The intelligence that created us does not come from the heart or the brain." Margaret looked around the room, unhurried. "How do we enter into a relationship with this creative intelligence we've had from the beginning? We'll need to access a wider frame. One that allows for a new capacity to see and to change."

All my experiences in the medical system were about rooting out problems, fixing what was broken, medicating what was symptomatic. This approach suggested life wasn't teetering between disease and health but actually contained some coherence and breathability; one whole organism, a me with a range of expressions. Margaret wasn't asking me to bypass what was wrong but suggesting that amid the disease a blueprint of my deep health still hummed along.

What if all is well? landed like a small seed in my chest, planted the idea that there was a way of trusting myself—my health, even—despite convincing evidence that I was deeply not okay. This didn't relieve my symptoms or erase my frustrations, but it did crack something open; instead of a binary separating the parts of me that were well and the sick parts I'd hoped to wall off, it suggested that *well* wasn't a land I could get back to but one in which I already dwelled. After so many years of trying to prove I was fine, it felt thrilling to listen for health without denying the reality of my illness. But most convincingly, regarding my life as a subtle and expansive field of possibilities *felt better*. The tendrils began to green up my ways of seeing and trusting myself so that I felt less braced and more inhabited. What creative ignitions might I discover if I wasn't waiting for some better, healthier, less painful version of myself? Lots, it turned out.

I want to take care here, to say clearly that there is an art to centering on what is well without denying or dismissing what very much isn't. I will not be refusing medication or the advice of practitioners because all is well and my self-trust is robust. I won't shame myself or anyone else for seeking any pathway toward healing, and I would not be alive without medical intervention and care. Period. Full stop. The choices we make to feel better are deep and deeply personal.

Nor is this a gratitude practice, a way of insisting on the bright side, or an embrace of "things happen for a reason." Folks who have experienced rupture or illness know how often and quickly the world asks us to grow through our pain, to make something beautiful or useful out of the awful. We know the quiet blame that comes with expectations that we *get better already* and the disappointments when we do not. I am still a person who lives with disease and its often terrible symptoms. But reclaiming myself at scale makes space to organize around the parts that nourish alongside the parts that pain; it helps me see myself whole. And I am very interested in accessing that wholeness that gives us back our humanity and makes flourishing possible.

Way back on that autumn evening, this was planted too: If we dip into this more expansive field where all is well, what else might we find? Could voice, writing, and expression also be a way of fortifying our health and accessing our deep intelligence? Perhaps the very origins of this book are there on that September night, meeting a radically different way of occupying a life.

TRASHCANS AND HURRICANES / EXPLAINING BIODYNAMIC CRANIOSACRAL THERAPY TO AN EIGHT-YEAR-OLD

If you are in my line of work, there is a thing that happens at parties and barbecues: Someone asks what you do and as soon as you say the words *biodynamic craniosacral therapist*, you've . . . lost them. Biodynamic craniosacral. It's such a mouthful that it buries itself.

Then one day on the way to school, as we passed by wild turkeys and frozen fields, my daughter, Nora—eight years old at the time—asked a question from the backseat that got to the heart of this problem.

"But what do you really do? When you work it looks like . . . nothing."

I completed my foundation training with Dr. Kate Klemer in 2018. Every day I saw how powerful the work was, but I had not cracked this particular code: how to simply explain what it is. Because an eight-year-old? She doesn't want to hear about the relational field and down regulation; she couldn't care less about cerebrospinal fluid and the sphenobasilar junction. And if you can't help a kid understand what you do in practical language, can you really explain what you do?

I took a breath. "Well . . . " How could I convey the idea of energy? "Let's say there's a hurricane, and it blows over the trashcan. It just topples over and starts sliding across the street. What would happen if you walked out in the middle of the hurricane and stood it back up?"

"It would knock over again."

"Right. And again, and again. As long as the hurricane's blowing, the trashcan's falling over." I checked the rearview mirror to make sure she was still with me. "But, what if you could talk directly to the hurricane? What if you could understand energy—forces that are everywhere and invisible, but not always as loud as a hurricane—and help the hurricane start to calm. Then what would happen to the trashcan?"

"It would just stay put." We were getting somewhere. *Energy precedes matter* is a fundamental principle of biodynamics. If we talk to the underlying patterns, we influence everything else, trashcans included.

"And what if we zoomed right in—on this steering wheel, or my bag here or your leg. What would we see?"

"Dust." This was . . . so true. It was February, after all. I kept going.

"Yes. And if we zoomed in *even* further than that? Just kept zooming in and in?"

"Atoms."

"Yes!" I was trying not to get overly excited. "Okay, and if we zoom in on the atoms, what do we see?"

"Electrons?"

"Right! We've got these electrons spinning round and round protons and neutrons. We've actually got—when we get right down to this atomic zoom level—we've actually got much more space than stuff. If we focus on the space, we influence the stuff." *We are more space than matter.* In this practice, we're less interested in the conditional adaptations than the health that underlies it all. We focus on what is well, on what organizes health. My daughter seemed to be getting this.

"So, you speak the language of energy? Like, you know the words and sentences to talk to energy?" Kids are quick.

"Yes. But language is a lot about listening. You know how there are certain people you want to talk to and certain people you . . . don't?" I parodied an awkward adult to show what I meant, "'Do you like school, little girl?' We want to listen in a way that makes you comfortable enough to come out of your shell, so that we can have a real conversation and maybe shift things together." *Establishing resonance.*

So there, in five minutes, is a beginner's guide to biodynamic craniosacral therapy: trashcans, hurricanes, dust, listening. Maybe I'll try that at the next barbecue.

BODY/LANGUAGE

Biodynamic craniosacral therapy (BCST) began to train me in how to hold space that was engaged but not watchful or scrutinizing. Although from the outside a session looked very quiet and uneventful—a client would lie on a table, a practitioner placed their hands gently on an area for a while, the client got up—this feeling of being accompanied in what practitioners call *a safe relational field* (what we might also call co-regulation) was profound. I learned to recognize the quiet processes inside a session that were the hallmarks of nervous system healing: settling, moments of activation, reorganizing, changes in state, needs for space, changes in pacing.

Surprisingly, although BCST is a body-based, hands-on therapy, it offered me something I didn't know I was missing: language. Language for actually inhabiting a body. Because while we have lots of ways to describe a body *from the outside*, describing a body from the inside can be remarkably difficult, at turns both awkward and inadequate.

Early in our lives, when we fall down or scrape our knees, most of us English speakers learn to say *it* hurts. We do not usually say *I* hurt. From the beginning, the landscape of our bodied experience is mapped to an impersonal outside. No wonder that naming and claiming language that describes us from within as a living, breathing, moment-to-moment unfolding is something most of us don't know how to do. Let's take a moment to try:

Pause and notice what your body is feeling right now. How would you describe it? Without guiding questions to find the way in, most people have a very hard time with this exercise. *Fine, I guess?* Others go right into stories and feelings. *I'm hungry, late for work, my stomach hurts—was it the cream cheese? I love cream cheese. I remember this one time . . .*

If we're listening from the organism of the body, we need to let all that sophistication go. It's a bit like opening your eyes underwater or taking off your glasses if you're near sighted. The view is blurry and undefined, so you'll have to recruit other ways of gathering information: the temperature, textures, colors, sense of pace, and movement. Areas of your body that light up in response. Images that come drifting through. Our minds are so very good at planning, analyzing, and future forecasting. But if we are going to invite our nervous systems along for the ride, we want to recognize a different kind of intelligence, a thinking body. As you drop beneath judgment and meaning-making, you actually tune toward a more present read of what's happening in the right now. Whether or not we're consciously practicing, this awareness is always humming in the background. As you're reading this, some part of you is noticing sound, room tone, mood, feeling, safety.

Listening this way takes practice but yields treasure. When you're not chasing down an explanation for *why* this is here or *when* it will stop, or what you ate/did/messed up to get this way, everything shifts. We drop into what I think of as nervous system wisdom and its less precise, deeply intelligent way of noticing the unfolding now. This getting into the body opens up new pathways to being with our whole selves.

Here in the present moment where we haven't seen the movie already, we get to be surprised. We get to wonder. We get to explore awareness beneath cognition, which, if we are writing, will enliven our language with freshness, animating scene, self, emotion, memory, and discovery.

Practice

THE VIEW FROM UNDERWATER

When I'm in an autoimmune flare, I can get a little lost excavating why I ended up here. I want so much to lay out the pieces like a jigsaw, or a map. *See here, how you overextended? And this time, when you allowed yourself whipped cream, your secret nemesis?*

But sometimes, symptoms defy explanation, and my attempts to ascribe order, meaning, and reason actually come in on the channel of *how I screwed this all up again.* Which can feel like quite the pileup: I'm flaring, and now, in ways I can't explain, it's also my fault.

Sometimes it's kinder to drop interpretation and be as direct as I can: *I am exhausted. I hurt. I'm thirsty.*

These observations don't help explain how I got here, but they do bring me to the present moment where I might meet my actual needs and relinquish some of those harsh judgments (rather than, say, imagining a fantastical time where I did all the things to prevent this). This direct, kind witness can be a balm for chronic illness as it can for depression, grief, for all the mysterious pains that visit us when they do.

And to be clear, this isn't a call for ignorance or silent withstanding. Treatment, support, and education are crucial—we need our practitioners and our teachers, our networks of care and information. Only that, in our rush to analyze, we can distance ourselves from life as it's being lived. In this practice, we're dropping why questions in favor of direct observation that meets us with kindness and immediacy.

Engage the Body

Take a moment to notice the scene around you. Let your gaze be sharp, precise. Then, let your vision go soft. If you wear glasses, you might remove them, or imagine that you're seeing the scene underwater—blurry, moving. Instead of focusing outward, see if you can let the scene arrive in your awareness from here.

Hear the sound of your breath, feel the way your limbs hang. Notice textures, areas of the body, smells, feeling, tingles, distractions. Are there images or metaphors that come to mind here? How does your sense of distance shift? What becomes interesting? Personally, I notice my attention and body soften. My inner dialogue sounds more like: *My breath loves to be slow. I'm interested in the shaft of sun falling from the skylight, warmth on my right shoulder, dots of color in the cup full of markers.*

Write

Now it's your turn. Rather than the keen perception of your eyes, see if you might listen from your whole body. What colors, textures, and temperatures do you notice?

Deepen

Pause. What's it like to let your noticing roam in this new way? Disorienting? Fascinating? Confusing?

FIRST WORKSHOP

Before I led my first workshop, I had these ideas about embodied writing swirling around in my head, this wild yet simple practice I wanted to share with others. But would they get it? Enjoy it? Did it even make sense outside of my own experience? I met up with my trusted friend Sage to put language to the idea.

"Your mind tracks forward, right?" I began. "And your emotions keep a catalog of every insult and injury of the past, but what if you got into your body, right here, in present time, and then you wrote? What if you interrupted your same old stories and let your body help locate new ones?"

"That," they said. "Do that." And offered their studio as a place we could meet—a former real estate office with dark carpeting, a makeshift herbal apothecary in the corner, and a light-up sign that spelled L-O-V-E.

I pulled together a flyer with a photo of a boat in the fog and a description. It read:

"What happens when you combine vital, embodied writing with deep listening? Join us for a daylong retreat to nourish our creative selves. Blending meditation and gentle movement with writing exercises and (optional) sharing, we'll explore what happens in our writing when we invite our whole selves into the room."

I walked around town, tacking flyers up in yoga studios, health food stores, cafés where the bulletin boards were pockmarked and crowded with news of vegan potlucks and punk rock shows. I sent emails, created online posts. I was sure no one would understand what I was offering, let alone relinquish a Saturday to try it.

When the day arrived, I pulled up in front of Sage's studio two hours early. What if people didn't show up? What if they did? Either way, I needed plenty of time to set up. One full side of the space featured storefront windows that faced the street, and I wanted to make the room comfortable and inviting. A place we might let loose in the writing. I unloaded my overstuffed car, carrying in items one by one: a giant bag of colorful rubber balls in all sizes, meditation cushions in shades of eggplant, a potted fern, chocolates, almonds, and tea. In the center of the carpet I unfolded a small square cloth, and placed on it flowers, snacks, a lit candle, and a river stone.

Finally, I laid out my only truly essential tools, the ones that had carried me through every chapter of life. Notebook and pen. Though I'd dabbled a bit in fancy journals and ballpoint pens, I had come to rely on the smooth, fresh lines of whatever CVS stocked in its stationary aisle and a cheap Bic round point. The ability of these objects to disappear was the point. Tools so unremarkable and unpretentious that they let my words emerge with no preoccupation of performance. Like garden clothes, these were objects I used when I intended to get messy, to reach my hands in the dirt of life, seeding something I hoped might grow or nourish or make the place more beautiful.

Improbably, and to my surprise, delight, and trepidation, people started arriving. Sue, who was in her seventies, buoyant, folding herself neatly into a cross-legged position on the floor, lithe as a yoga instructor. (She was, in fact, a yoga instructor.) Deb, dark haired and deep eyed, exuding a serious warmth. One by one they assembled, creating a constellation of personalities that—once formed—we couldn't imagine any other way.

I folded my hands behind my back to hide my nervous shaking. Pulled out a lesson plan I'd written and overwritten: six single-spaced pages of notes. Took a breath. Took in the chatter.

"Can I sit here?"

"I signed up, but I don't actually know what we're doing. Sounded interesting."

"Could you pass the chocolate?"

Five hours. I had five hours to try and convey this thread I'd been holding, this bizarre conviction that creativity and the body belong together, belong to each other. That for too long, we'd separated these parts, pretending they weren't inextricably linked. That if we could open this conversation together, between our bodies and our language, we might access something deep and true.

Sitting there, waiting for the workshop to begin, reminded me of a job I'd had at nineteen, working in the Tusayan Museum on the Grand Canyon's South Rim. Every day, I'd lead tourists on a circular path, reciting facts I barely knew to folks who wouldn't remember them. "Did you know that piñon pine trees' nuts contain an astounding 190 calories per handful?" I'd exclaim. "That's more than a bag of M&M's!" But if the visitors asked about anything outside of my memorized script, I stuttered awkwardly.

Now here I was again, pretending to guide a group of mostly strangers through a practice I was just discovering myself. Sure, I was older and more experienced, but the fear of being found out as a newbie brought me right back to that museum of eroded relics. No wonder the metaphor that kept surfacing was *ruin*. As in: Will I have ruined their afternoon? Ruined any affection they had for writing, or movement, or me?

Maybe this was the secret legacy of being a child of immigrants. In some quiet way I was waiting for the authorities to leap out—from the museum gift shop, the herbal apothecary in the corner—and demand I show my papers. Justify the ruse. Maybe this is the legacy of anyone who steps off the path to try something new and untested, bracing to get called out or have permission revoked. Anticipating the question: *Who gives you the right?*

But that is not what happened.

"I'm here because I have a young child at home and I just . . . miss myself and my songwriting," said Penelope, a musician.

Maya stretched out on a rubber ball I'd brought to work the back body and let out such a satisfied moan that we all broke our seriousness and got down to it, rolling, softening, exploring.

Anna, a graceful acupuncturist in her sixties, wrote about the lavender fields back home in Argentina and wept. We all did.

Putting my props away at the end of the day, I thought how impostor syndrome can come in so many flavors. Not only when we're offering something new, but even in the privacy of our own lives, a kind of merciless questioning can creep in: *How do I justify trying something so frivolous and unnecessary? Why make time for whimsy when so many other things need my attention?* It takes courage to step off the track and try something unfamiliar. But when we do we discover how utterly worthwhile and meaningful it is to stretch in these new ways. Essential, actually.

Everyone who attended that day had made the decision to dignify their creative embodiment with devoted time. They brought a kind of willingness, and by the end of those hours, we had become something together, a coherence borne of listening, and moving, and stepping into the unknown. What we discovered in that room, that I've witnessed in hundreds of workshops since, and that I hope to share with you in these pages, is how these simple elemental ingredients shifted something deep within. Regardless of the conditions we carried, we found a way to show up in our fullness together and tell new stories about our unfolding lives.

FIRST PERSON

Creative Energy Is Healing Energy

Arly Scully is a massage therapist and writer who lives in Portland, Maine. Embodied writing helps her connect her body to her body of work.

The summer of 2021 I was having a really difficult time connecting with Muse, with my body, with my work. (Which is to say: I was having a really difficult time connecting with *myself*.) Vaccines had been released—yay science!—but the world had changed. In a COVID-oriented world, space took on a new meaning. How we interact with bodies—our own and those of others—had greatly shifted. As a licensed massage therapist with thousands of (hu)man hours logged and a lifelong storyteller, I was petrified that I might have lost the ability to drop into the containers that allow me to connect the two loves of my life: the human body and the words we use to name and claim our experiences.

And then Johanna showed up in my inbox, offering an invitation to a somatic writing workshop called "Writing Ourselves Awake." This was a virtual offering, and I'll admit I was skeptical about what might happen via Zoom. But I also opened the email and said out loud, "Yes. I need this." So without a ton of attachment to the outcome, I signed up. Logged on. And let myself see what might happen.

There it was. There *I* was. Over the series of a few weeks, exploring these somatically rich and permission-based prompts, I found myself fully connecting my body to my body of work. Surprise, delight, relief, connection—this is what I found when I worked in this new way.

Over the past few years I have visited and revisited these prompts, both in communion with Johanna and on my own. And each time I am amazed to find that my words have a weight to them that is simply not present when I use nonsomatic prompts from others. There is a "thereness" to the prose and poetry that shows up after working through the suggestions and guidance Johanna has created for us. When I work with these invitations, I'm far better able to show up for my body and my writings. (Which is to say: I'm far better able to show up for myself.)

Embodied writing reminded me that creative energy *is* healing energy.

How (Not) to Listen to a Body

BEFRIENDING THE INNER ALLY

2007. It was getting weird over here in the tea aisle, where I had picked up and set down a box of chamomile tea five times, pausing between each gesture to hold the box to my sternum, close my eyes, and wait.

Nothing.

This one? A rooibos? Or this? I tried mint, ginger, Earl Grey—I had no idea what I was doing. Recently diagnosed with an autoimmune disease, this was one more in a series of bafflements.

Around me, a din of beeps from the register, a child's whine in the next aisle, a woman whose perfume bloomed out behind her.

A therapist had recommended this bizarre exercise as a way of practicing what she'd called *listening to your body*. The idea was to check in with what I actually wanted rather than an idea of what I wanted. To discern the opening affirmation that would signal a subtle yes, the quiet contraction of no. Go to the supermarket, she'd suggested, and spend some time practicing with a low-stakes choice.

But what did that even mean, listening to a body?

I was always saying yes when I meant no. I said yes to jobs, people, promises, engagements of all kinds. I said yes with a smile, intending, in all sincerity, to follow through.

But then my body would say something else, spinning out in outrageous and creative conflagrations—presentations I couldn't argue with: incontinence, blood, fevers, sores, exhaustion, stomach pain that left me howling on the floor or contorted over the toilet. My body screamed with an insistence that seemed to drown everything else out until, tearfully, I asked for a leave from grad school, from my job, from another project, from a party down the block, from, from, from.

So, clearly, my body was talking. But it felt crazy—*I* felt crazy—that I kept backing into decisions I only found my way out of by spectacularly coming apart.

I put back the chamomile, turned to the lower shelves of Tetley and Celestial Seasonings, the cheaper options, less adorned with promises. Maybe my body would find a way to feeling its yes through something more familiar and less expensive? This was harder than I'd expected.

Here in the early aughts, before nervous system care and embodiment were common terms, all I registered from my body was how thoroughly and totally it was getting in the way of my plans. Older me might sit young me down and ask plaintively, *It? It was getting in the way of your plans? Or you? How have you so depersonalized your body that these imaginary plans are realer to you than the howl you've just hidden in the staff bathroom? The abscess developing in your rectum?*

And younger me, I imagine, might answer, *Get lost. I have things to do.*

Go on and try, older me would say. *I'll wait.*

Because there will be a moment, several years into this disease, when the aperture begins to open on something else, and I'll get a first glimpse of what listening to a body might mean.

It happened at the end of a week I'd spent with kind older friends I refer to as my fairy godparents. Deb and Bill fed my voracious steroidal appetite with roasted chicken, pork loin, good cheese. They offered acupuncture treatments, walked with me on the beach as I wept. I had my own room with soft sheets and windows that looked down the mountains toward the sea. Their care was so generous and abundant that, bathing in this elixir, it unsettled me out of numbness and confronted me with my true state: exhausted, unrecognizable. Steroids had bloated my face into a swollen pancake; blood loss had made me anemic and uncertain. Suddenly I could not summon the impulse that pushed me hard enough to erase these realities.

One night I dreamed that I was lashed to the bottom rim of a teetering gyroscope, each rotation scraping my body across the concrete, cutting me open. The image startled me awake: How had it come to this? I'd been so focused on the scenery going round and round—*the things I had to do*—that I'd ignored the cost. The truth was so horrifying I could only admit it in a whisper: *I've been living as if I don't matter.* I felt as if someone had suddenly switched on the lights, and I was squinting at a reality I did not know how to navigate. If I wasn't steering myself by what the world required of me, how was I to move? What would life even look like?

And then, on my way home, when the plane's fasten seatbelt light came on, I heard a clear, distinct voice: *Sweetheart, you can still use the bathroom if you need it. You just get yourself what you need right now.*

I looked around, startled. No one else had heard this voice, it seemed to be coming from inside of me.

The voices that told me to push through, to get over it, that asked why I was so insistent on not getting better were familiar to me. But this was new, not something I could have conjured if I tried. And yet there it was, this strange inner ally.

I have a hunch the flight attendants would have had some fairly strong objections to my jumping up at the moment of liftoff to declare my entitlement to the bathroom. But the possibility that something within might advocate for me was electric, radical. My life as something that mattered—more even than the responsibilities I had or the commitments I'd made—began to change an old way of operating.

This is what I'd missed back in the supermarket, waiting for a mystery reaction to those tea boxes: Listening to your body is not a parlor trick; it isn't necessarily a body sensation at all, not a code to crack or an intuitive tingle at the back of the neck. If I wanted to listen, I would have to, as my therapist said, *do* different. I would have to choose my own side, grant myself enough permission to follow an impulse that came from who knows where. Not dress up my impatience with an exercise in "listening" that waited for me to have a bodily response already, but rather I needed to be willing to dignify my not knowing with lots of space.

It would be a long time before I understood that creating this kind of space for myself was an act of love.

When I was trying to "listen to my body," what I really wanted was to figure out what was wrong, to stop the flaring, to get my body to follow the plans I had for my life.

If I'm honest, what I wanted was compliance.

If I'm honest, I still want compliance. You may still want this too. But because we have to, perhaps we could settle for this inner kindness that offers us permission to live in the bodies we actually have. In part II we'll try out new ways of orienting to what's right here and language that feels authentic. My hope is that as you practice this listening and writing you begin to discover a way back in, not to compliance but to yourself.

PART II

The Check-In

Settling, arriving. Learning to listen from a body.

In part II, we turn from guided settling toward checking in with how we are on this day and moment, developing tools and techniques that help us listen from our bodies in the here and now. We'll begin to invite deeper settling and discover new tools that get directly into specific body sites.

WHAT LANGUAGE CAN DO

Back in the early days of my autoimmune disease, before my medical records took up an entire file cabinet, I found myself constantly befuddled by the language of the medical field.

When medication after (ridiculously costly) medication didn't work, I was told I had failed them. My medical paperwork classified my colon as "noncompliant." And when I called the nurse to say I was too weak and inflamed to eat, she told me she'd make a note that my situation was emergent.

"Emergent?" I asked. "Hasn't it already emerged fully? Are we waiting for something else to happen?"

"No," She sighed. "As in *emergency*."

Oh. This was not my kind of poetry.

Because language mattered to me. Language has always mattered to me. I was the kid who stood on the periphery of the room soaking up words. I kept journals before I could write, scribbling approximated proto-letters. As an adult, part of my work is to listen for the dynamics underneath what is said, feeling for sensation and belief. So I recognized what was happening; these words pretended neutrality, but they told me everything about how the medical system regarded a body like mine: deviant, failing. Uninhabited.

And yes, I get the utility of reducing a body to its pathologies in a system that's supposed to fix them, but it felt like such a missed opportunity. Because words can also be a source of great, enlivening support.

Resonant language—in poetry or story or lyric—creates recognition and repair. When I'm feeling overwhelmed by the terrible, words are a map to what matters. There are treasures there, secret instructions.

Consider the word *solace,* which comes from the Latin *solari,* to console. But *solari* derives from the Greek *hilaros,* meaning "cheerful," what you might recognize as the source of hilarious.

Inside *solace*, this truth: To get through the difficult, we need both care and humor. Which, if you've experienced illness or grief, you likely already know. Overserious sympathy can sap our reserves. But a well-landed, irreverent joke? Real solace.

If you listen, you might start to recognize the places where language lifts and connects. Like a video meet up with friends titled, "World is ending / friendship is mending." Or the unreasonable joy I get from the memes my sisters send, equal parts rallying and ridiculous ("How can you make jokes at a time like this?!" "Sir, that dark sense of humor is a load-bearing structure.")

For me, reclaiming my body back from the medical field also meant finding language that described me from the inside. It's what led me to develop an embodied writing practice, to this book you are holding. Because language can guide our attention to wonder, grief, absurdity, the ribald, the beautiful, each other. To a place where we *celebrate* our noncompliance.

And language can also help us locate what's true in our lives and bodies, so long as we *start where we are*. In our workshops, arriving and checking in are essential parts of the process; when we name the specificities of this day, this breath, or this mood, we're practicing language that is alive and authentic. Here in part II, we're learning to listen from a whole self, granting ourselves abundant permission for trying something new, and discovering tools that get directly into specific body sites.

Outside my window, an early spring cluster of white and purple crocuses. Now *this*, I think, is emergent. Life is emergent. So are you.

CLUELESS

When I was twenty-three, I moved to the Costa Rican cloud forest to teach English and social studies to middle schoolers at a small bilingual Quaker school. I had very little clue of what I was doing except that I knew I wanted to get as far away from New York as possible, and that a small village in the tropics felt about right. In preparation, I read a large stack of books on education and team building, I mapped out units and lesson plans, and I bought a bag of beautiful scraps of paper: tiny slips of zebra prints, flowers laced through with gold thread, handmade layers of blue fiber. In between study units and activities, my plan was to leave notes for my students, quietly noticing their brave acts or kindnesses, and tuck these into their desks.

I bumbled through so many of my days. The 3D maps I had students craft out of flour and water turned to disgusting, gloppy piles of mush in the cloud forest humidity, destroying mountains and valleys kids had spent hours making. The marshmallow eating contest I thought would build camaraderie ended in at least two severe cases of indigestion. Undeterred, each morning I climbed the dirt road to the little school on the mountain, a backpack stuffed with lesson plans and notes, a packed lunch of sandwiches and fruit. I was absolutely making it up as I went along, but I was also falling in love with those kids and felt determined to win them over.

Not everyone was a fan.

One boy, a red-headed ten-year-old named Ben, did not love school, which got in the way of more important endeavors, like soccer and not-school. He frequently scowled when I introduced new activities or rushed through whatever time-wasting assignments I'd concocted. I lobbed everything I had in an attempt to crack his shell—jokes, stories, asides. Notes of praise and recognition written on scraps from my stash of fancy paper. Nothing.

Months went by. And then one day, partway through a unit on Norse mythology, I noticed that Ben's left hand was balled up around . . . something. He carried it around all day, this thing poking out of his small fingers, a little piece of paper.

One of the notes I'd left him. Utterly unacknowledged, but evidently important. When we cleaned out his desk at the end of the year, I found my notes crumpled and kept, his desk a secret stash. Tiny records of how he'd shown up and been noticed.*

Trying something new is awkward. Doubly so when we have no reassurance that we're doing it right. We call into the chasm, and it is echoless; put ourselves out there and endure the nothing that comes back.

But making meaningful change means *we haven't been here before.* Which is another way of saying *we do not know what we're doing.* We cannot skip this vital, terrible, awkward step. Forgive me if I am overly emphasizing this, but it feels important to say here at the beginning: You do not need to know how to do this.

Perfectionism wants to skip to the end, get it right. Perfection is tethered to a notion of goodness we don't own for ourselves; it insists on benchmarks that can be measured on a single line. And it is supremely impatient, wanting things done already.

Contrary to what you've maybe trained your whole life for up until now, in this embodied writing practice we lower our expectations down, down, down until they are low enough so that we can play here on the floor with ourselves. So that we can get loose and—here is the kicker—stop caring so much about the recognition we receive in return. Not knowing pops us off that taut perfectionist line of right or wrong and into something much richer, more interesting, and messy.

But this is also a story of staying. Of surrendering to an orientation that is willing to be in loving—or at least unhurried—connection. Despite how annoying I was or how thankless Ben seemed, we did not give up on each other. I pulled on a thread, and he pulled back. Transformations are built of this stuff; if we can stay in connection through discomfort, *something else* gets to happen. And at the root

* When he graduated college, Ben sent me a kind note of his own, reflecting on our time together in the classroom. He's now a deeply loving partner and father who's channeled that wonderful defiance into advocacy.

of this practice, we are opening to that something else that lets more of us into our lives.

Friends, we haven't been here before. So if you can bring real gentleness to doing something unfamiliar—like getting into your body to write, like wandering a tea aisle to listen more deeply, like a ridiculous attempt to connect with someone—you might feel the carapace of trying slide away, easing you into softer ways of being. Let's not skip to the end, that bodiless fantasy, but be willing to stay here in the messy middle, clueless, dropping love notes for our future selves.

Practice

AWKWARD BEGINNINGS

In this practice we want to begin to let your creativity / nervous system / body know that we are practicing in the spirit of being a true beginner; *not* knowing is welcome here.

Engage the Body

Allow yourself to get still and quiet. Let your attention wander to a time or place when you wanted something and heard crickets. Perhaps this was a relationship or a job, a recognition, a shift in life of some kind.

See if you can get quiet enough to feel the tug of your own wanting, perhaps you might also detect the absence of a callback. See if you can notice how this feels from the body's awareness. What parts get activated, pushed, compressed? What does this impatience feel like?

Then, begin to notice the spaces that are quieter, that surround this urgency and tug. See if you can drop out of the timeline of frustration and into a wider space, a longer arc. Is there any new information you collect when you're not gripping here? Can you make space for mystery?

Do you feel any difference between expectant waiting and simply not knowing?

Write

Imagine you might locate yourself within the spaces that feel easier and less taut or frustrated. What do these places of ease have to say to the more difficult places? Perhaps they might offer some patience or perspective, some familiarity with being a beginner?

PRESENCE WITHOUT SCRUTINY

Our family learned that new neighbors had moved in next door when seven-year-old Z showed up in our driveway one afternoon, big brown eyes and curls, and a gap where his left front tooth used to be. He met my daughter and the other neighborhood kids in the way children do. Effortlessly, the game was already on: They were pulling each other on the zip line, someone was asking if everyone knew the rules for toilet tag.

And then, twenty minutes after they said goodbye, there was a knock at the door. "Hey," said Z, without preamble. "I made this mask for you." He held out a rectangular piece of paper with two holes cut out, something like a flag drawn on the front, pencil sketches of a Pacman ghost, lightning bolts, a smiling shovel.

"Oh," I said, "is this a character you've created?"

"No. I just made a mask." He turned over the paper. "See how I put some tape here between the eyes to reinforce it." And then he took off across the lawn.

"Thanks!" We called after him.

Much has been written on the early creative injuries that stunt our making as we grow into adulthood. Harsh criticism, detached disinterest, and even meaningless praise—each, in its way, takes the seedling of making and sets it under the hot lamp of evaluation; it unhomes creativity from the body and demands it live in the colorless metric of how good it is or isn't. It's not only the creative process that suffers in this dynamic. Working with clients, I've noticed that if an agenda has been set by the practitioner, the teacher, or even by ourselves, something is snuffed out. *Have to* has a way of shutting down any process of discovery.

Standing there, Z's mask in hand, I was struck by the giddy magic of what Z had just done and how I'd seen it before. I recognized the same feeling with embodied writing participants, teens I'd taught how to make radio stories, and toddlers.

Being seen matters. When we're ready, we often *want* to share our work. This creating and being witnessed feeds us on some fundamental level. We do not, however, love a microscope. We want the seeing to be spacious. The creative process needs space, mystery, a little less reason. Rather than a direct stare or a demand for explanation, we'd prefer you stand off to the side, offering soft, oblique attention.

We want presence, not scrutiny.

Engaged, compassionate witnessing is why reading and sharing are an essential part of our embodied writing practice, but critique is not. In workshops, after someone shares their writing, we reflect back what we hear, echoing the parts that moved us. We don't bring a corrective lens to what's nascent. Even if you're practicing on your own, your notebook is its own potent form of witness, a record of what you made, thought, saw. And it's why I recommend that you read your words aloud, so you can feel them spoken, made audible.

Part of the work of this book is to help you care for your nervous system, that complex inner web of responding to life. But "nervous system," much like "embodied," gestures to such a wide range of applications that it can lose meaning. So, rather than getting into a technical description of the ventral vagal nerve or exploring the sympathetic and parasympathetic systems, I'd invite you to employ this simple and direct frame: a perceptive and deep-feeling child, offering you the gift of their creativity. Do not stare, crowd, or ask why. Show up with tenderness.

Standing there, I thought that next time I get stuck in self-doubt and critique I will remember this gap-toothed boy showing me exactly what to do. Just the next thing. Just the thing that tugs, and then gift it away, without thought or explanation, apology or excuse. *I made this for you.* And in that act, I could be generous, be unthinking. I could stand on the porch of someone new and let myself be seen.

Practice BREATH

You are breathing.

It's a truth so self-evident we might forget the magnitude of the miracle. Every moment of every day you are drawing in and releasing breath, feeding your cells, moving carbon dioxide out and oxygen in. Of course, breath isn't only anatomical. Breath is also a great teacher in one of our body's deep truths: We're designed to move. Like tides, like moods, or the phases of the moon, we expand and contract, let go and begin again. Breath is also a magnificent proxy for the nervous system, because it echoes the themes we've been exploring around scrutiny as a flow-stopper. If you've ever tried to follow the instruction *pay attention to your breath*, you've likely noticed that direct attention can turn this otherwise effortless action stilted and effortful.

Deepening our relationship to breath gives us tools for recognizing some of the places we've gotten stuck. Are we holding our breath? Do we feel so overextended that we crave a fresh inhalation? Or a release of exhalation? Perhaps we need a reminder to let go and begin again.

In this practice, we sink into the wisdom of *just breathing* and practice *not* effort.

Engage the Body

Either seated or lying down, take a few minutes to simply breathe; inhale through the nose on a slow count of six, visualizing filling up from the bottom to the top of the lungs. As you exhale, empty out in reverse, from top to bottom, on a count of six. Spend a few moments afterward simply noticing.

Write

The space I need . . .

Deepen

As you bring your attention toward your breath, what do you notice? Explore what *breath tells me . . .*

FIRST PERSON

Discovering Lungs

Tessa Greene O'Brien is a painter who swims and writes on the coast of Maine.

I was well into my thirties when I realized that I perpetually hold my breath. During an embodied writing class Johanna asked me, with gentleness and the ever-present touch of humor in her voice; "Do you, um, breathe?" We both laughed, and then maybe I cried a little, realizing that breathing could be more than just panicky gulps "as needed."

In the same memorable workshop, we were lying in a circle on our backs and connecting with our breath. As this was a new concept for me, my mind wandered and I began to picture a tiny LEGO-like version of myself traveling down my esophagus with the breath, arriving in the chamber of my lungs. LEGO-me strolls around, taking in the warm and dimly lit space. The walls are curved, and the room is furnished oddly like the bear den on the Celestial Seasonings Sleepytime tea box. It feels somehow spacious and cozy at the same time, and LEGO-me patted the walls affectionately; my lungs registered as home.

This breathing exercise is followed by a ten-minute writing prompt where I record the visualization. In reading it back, I am entertained by my own imagination, tickled to have formed a new pathway in my brain by connecting movement to language. Through writing and breathwork over the years since, I have now mapped my whole body's interior through the yellow plastic visor goggles of tiny LEGO-me, who has traveled on waves of my own breath deep into my toes, the backs of my quads, the space between my shoulders, and the crown of my skull.

STOP MAKING SENSE

Fresh out of college in 1999, I moved to New York City and took a job at a nonprofit organization that worked to reform the city's public schools. Each week, I rode the subway to different districts to attend conferences of school principals, noting if their schools were following state standards.

Perhaps a pause here to appreciate how laughable and embarrassing this scenario is: A twenty-two-year-old evaluating teachers and principals with decades of experience. Teachers and principals who had lived through enough Department of Education trends to know they would outlast this one too. Nevertheless, there I was with a clipboard and binder, taking notes and looking for evidence of things like *Student work is displayed in public spaces.* I understood none of it. Not the standards, not the conferences, not my choice of city or apartment or job.

I developed a strange verbal tick. "Oh," I'd say, nodding along to my supervisor, "That makes sense." To the principal explaining the posters on the walls. To my friends talking about their relationship problems. To my boyfriend describing his latest art project. "That makes sense."

Until my beloved friend Sepideh, who always tells me the truth, snapped at me one day. "What the hell is going on, Jonesy? You keep saying 'that makes sense' to nothing that makes sense! Are you even hearing the words?" No, no I wasn't. I was becoming a kind of empty shell, nodding along. Agreeable and vacant.

None of it made sense, but if I let in this truth I'd also have to acknowledge that none of this—the job, city, relationship—was working. I'd have to admit that I didn't have it together, which felt like a failure I couldn't cop to. I had no real signs of disease yet, but a small fissure was already beginning to form between what I presented on the outside and how I actually felt within.

If you'll allow me a brief digression . . .

In Stockholm there's a museum built to house the *Vasa*, an elaborate seventeenth-century royal warship. On its maiden voyage, not 1,400 yards from shore, a small puff of wind started the boat listing to port, and it promptly filled with water and sank to the bottom of the harbor. To be raised, nearly fully intact, hundreds of years later.

What caused the sinking remains a topic of great controversy: too little ballast to steady the ship, extra decks that created a top-heavy vessel, lower gun ports open in maiden-voyage salute. But this fact remains: No one had the temerity to tell the king how disastrously unseaworthy it was, which meant no one stopped the catastrophe. Ego made the thing susceptible in all the wrong ways.

I wonder if, in the museums of our lives, we'd all have these exhibitions of folly. Times when the stakes felt too high or our egos were too weak, and so we didn't name the truth but plowed ahead, declaring that these precarious decisions "made sense," only to be undone later by a crashing, sinking conflagration. We were so focused on what was happening above deck, the gilded bow, the sails shining in the wind, that we ignored the less visible gut feelings below. And so we set off, ignoring the very vessel that would make the whole journey possible.

Here in our explorations, we're pausing to note, with supreme gentleness, the places where we feel this schism between inside and outside, or the distance between what we felt and what we said or did. Doing so might help us tend to the ballast of our own ships, the supports below deck that aren't ornamented or shiny, but infinitely more honest, capacious, and rooted in what supports us through the storm. It's an approach that makes a profound kind of sense.

Practice

MUSEUM OF FOLLIES

Imagine you might create your own museum of follies. As the curator, please keep in mind that this is not a museum of blaming or shaming, and we won't be exhibiting moments that feel overwhelming or too tender. Instead, roam through the scenes of your life to collect artifacts and images of times and places that did not make sense, maybe creating interactive displays and placards to place around the room.

I can imagine a case featuring my sister's single precious lipstick, which I extended fully and then thoughtlessly capped. The title: *How could you? 1985.* In another, the hippy pants I borrowed for a weeklong meditation retreat but never properly learned to tie, thereby flashing the entire sangha. *Mistakes were made, 2000.* One wing of the museum would feature remedies and supplements and photographs of various attempts to quell the burning in my body: *I did the best I could at the time, 2003–.*

Engage the Body

As you roam through your own artifacts and images, notice how it feels in your body to visit these memories. What resources might you include to make the encounter more comfortable? Benches? A door to the beach? A slide that delivers you out of the past and into the current day? Feel free to be wildly inventive and deeply kind.

Write

A guided tour of my museum of follies . . .

A SHIFT BY DEGREES

Growing up, my father ran a sailing center on Boston Harbor, two blocks from our fourth-floor apartment in the North End. My sisters and I spent many of our summers oiling teak, prepping boats, and driving the launch for the center's large fleet of boats. But "ran a sailing center," doesn't really convey the degree to which my father knows oceans, boats, and wind, or how deeply this knowledge shaped my understanding of the world.

My dad can (and *has*, through a mid-Atlantic hurricane in the '70s) navigate his way across the Atlantic with only a sextant. He can patiently answer any question involving weather, planets, or math, which we regularly send his way: *Could you ride a bicycle on Mars? Explain the Gulf Stream.*

With this kind of rigor, it may come as no surprise that sailing trips were not ambling pleasure cruises but feats of speed and calculation. How precisely could we trim the sails; how quickly could we arrive?

My father used a divider and parallel rules to plot our course across giant navigational charts, then mapped it to a specific compass heading. Calculation complete, he'd call out to me at the helm.

"Jo!" he'd say, "steer 242." Gripping the tiller, I'd make subtle adjustments to keep the half orb of the compass centered on our heading.

I developed an early appreciation for how even the smallest, most undetectable shift can change an entire trajectory. When you're navigating across an ocean, a few degrees to the north could be the difference between, say, Miami and Halifax.

Turns out all of this nautical talk has surprising resonance in life. Like a compass, your nervous system knows that real growth happens by degrees: Whatever changes you incubate here, no matter how small or undetectable, set your course to a different land entirely—a place where other things are possible. But we cannot get there by leaping over the present and into some imagined future—Fiji, say, or a place where all trauma and illness have resolved—but by companioning ourselves in the journeying present, with its shifting weather and tides.

This can be a difficult thing to remember in the middle of a storm. In times of turmoil we tend to batten down the hatches and stay the course rather than shift our orientation. After all, didn't we make it this far doing it the same old way? We did, *and yet*. If we want to move to more habitable waters, we may need to change an approach that locks down in order to make it through. Despite how loud this moment is, remembering the longer arc of our unfolding life opens a different route. Small shifts incubate radical change. This seemingly slow approach is paradoxically the most efficient; the steady, subtle movements shift the whole vessel.

Craniosacral practitioner Susan Raffo writes that our work is to help folks "imagine just two cells wider than what today feels like. What if? What if?"[3] We aren't here to push an agenda or yank away patterns that got you this far. Instead, we practice a small deviation from where we've been pointing. A tiny, manageable shift. It's a subtle practice, but it changes everything.

Practice

SMALL SHIFTS

As you get ready to write, pause to notice if there are any microadjustments you could make toward comfort. Is it possible to work a little less hard to be right where you are? We often need a few moments to move from "No, I'm fine. Everything's fine" to "Actually, this elastic is pulling at my scalp. And my jeans are too tight, and truthfully my leg is falling asleep." Good. Noticing these small, quiet places of withstanding are portals to a new way of inhabiting our bodies in present time, and they begin to wake up our old ways of accommodating.

Which sounds grandiose—really? Loosening my belt is the gateway to change?—but once you start noticing the small discomforts you've been ignoring, you begin to notice the larger patterns of override and accommodation. I remember once mentioning to a therapist that a friend was coming for dinner, so I'd planned to make quiche. Although, I admitted, the cream-heavy meal would give me stomachaches for days.

"Wait," said the therapist. "Wait. Why are you choosing a thing that will hurt you? Why are we ignoring your body here?" And it helped me see a tiny, invisible thing I'd done for years, insisting oh, it's *fine* because I'd assumed a little pain, or actually a lot, was the cost of participation in the human field. It had never occurred to me that it didn't have to be this way. That this level of suffering was not a given. All this from plans for a quiche!

If we are making way for your actual shape, from the granularity of your posture to the needs of your digestion to the large decisions of life, we only need to start right here, letting these tiny shifts change everything.

While there are certainly pains and losses we can't make better, in this practice we're turning to the closer in impediments and discomforts that we *can* actually shift. We might call these microstressors; tending to these overlooked chafes can actually provide real relief by moving us out of a posture of withstanding and into something far more honest.

Engage the Body

Breathe deeply into your belly, getting loose, wide, and spacious. From here, see if you can notice what impedes your sense of ease. These may be physical discomforts (these pants: too tight!), house grouses (hello, pile of unfolded laundry), or general irritations (I said I would meet them tonight, and I truly do not want to). We're not looking to create a to-do list or control other people's behavior; we're simply noticing if there are small shifts we can attend to that might make life more breathable.

Write

What isn't actually fine? An invitation to be honest and unafraid in the accounting. Then, rereading your list, notice if there are any accommodations that feel easy to make, requests for help you might recruit, or rest you might take in simply acknowledging what's here.

Practice
FLUIDITY/WATER

I remember once when my daughter, Nora, was sick with a terrible cold. She had a sore throat, sniffles, and achy fever—the whole rotten lot. We were visiting my husband Jon's family in Florida for a precious break from Maine's winter, so the timing felt particularly cruel.

"Mama," she croaked, "I feel so bad. What if I feel this bad forever?" She was crying now, imagining the inevitable unending road of discomfort and missing out. My heart broke hearing this. Only seven years old and *forever* had landed with a thunk. Who among us does not know this terrible feeling, which seems to have a knack for visiting us precisely when things are at their worst?

I held her close, feeling her sweet, hot forehead. The acute symptoms were running their course, but I could see that her misery was also coming from this conviction that she was doomed to sickness forever. Parenting is so often shooting from the hip. Taking our best guess at what to offer. So I tried the first thing that came to mind.

"Well, lovey," I said. "You are sick and sad. But I promise: Things can change." We practiced together in the dark, saying it over and over: *Things can change.*

I've tried this in the midst of my own deep illness and despair, repeating the phrase even without faith in its veracity. *Things can change.* Listening at this register is actually fundamental to the work of tending a nervous system and inhabiting a body. When the impenetrable stuckness overwhelms, tuning toward the barest flutter of movement brings our attention somewhere else. Evidence, even minuscule, shows us that pulsing, breathing life is in here somewhere. That something else is possible.

Listening for fluidity helps me drop under familiar perseverations (when will I feel better? How? What do I do?) and remember that we are *fluid bodies*:

fundamentally changeable. Our bodies not only know water, they are mostly constituted by it. Before we emerged from the womb, we existed in a fluid world. This breath and this one and the next are all proof of fluidity, of movement, of change.

Engage the Body

Water is essential to life. Biochemist Albert Szent-Györgyi writes that "[w]ater is life's matter and matrix, mother and medium. There is no life without water."[4] Whether we encounter this fluid medium in our teacup, the shower, or breaking on the shore, it's an element that shows us life wants to move. Water whispers: *Everything changes. Spring comes again.*

Take a moment to recall an encounter with water (stream, lake, bath, rain etc.) that you enjoyed. See if you can call on some of your developing skills to notice your felt sense. What textures, temperatures, colors do you notice? What happens in your jaw, belly, mind as you sit beside this image?

Write

Sprint prompts are perfect for dropping right in to writing. Set your timer for three minutes and choose one of the following prompts. When you're done, reset the timer and try another. You might notice that each of these is a different way of encountering water, an element that moves.

- Snowflake
- Mug of tea
- Ice cube
- Ocean wave

Deepen

Water is a supremely sensorial element. Consider sounds of waves, drips, steam. Movements that whirl, flow, submerge. Experiences of floating, hydrating, bathing. Write about *a memory of water . . .*

ALIVE IN MY BONES

In my early thirties, I enrolled in an anatomy and physiology night class at the local community college. Twice a week, I'd pry Nora's toddler arms off my body, kiss Jon goodbye, and drive into town to learn about the world beneath the skin. I studied the textbooks and created giant stacks of flash cards to memorize: *Describe the protein pump. What are the muscles in the quadriceps group?* Nora, listening beside me at the kitchen table, would parrot back in her small singsong voice, "Biceps femoris! Semitendinosus! Semimembranosus!"

Textbooks are not known for lyrical evocative prose, but then I got to the chapter on connective tissue and started weeping.

My understanding had been wrong the whole time. Bone, I learned, *is* connective tissue. These weren't the brittle, desiccated relics that I found washed up on beaches. No. Inside their natural habitat of a body they were bendable, alive, electric. Not just bloody *but the place where blood is born.* At that very moment, the marrow in my bones was producing new blood cells, feeding my bloodstream through small capillaries.

Bones are constantly regenerative. Which means that while muscles carry the grudge of every strain and pull (*Remember that time you tweaked your shoulder in middle school?* your tendons seem to say. *We sure do . . .*), bones heal comparatively quickly. They're game to begin again. When Nora was eight, she broke her arm climbing a tree. Even as the mother in me was freaking out, the anatomy geek knew this injury would repair more easily than a muscle tear. (The sparkly pink cast helped too.)

Imagining bones this way made me rethink my notion of structure itself. Instead of a brittle rule, what if structure could be living, bendable support? Support that is *already* here for you, that has your back, literally and metaphorically. Reimagining my bones as supple rather than rigid invited a different kind of strength.

But the real reason I had such a weepy, visceral reaction to that textbook chapter was that it woke something in me, unsettled a kind of resignation I felt around my own autoimmune disease. On some level, I'd come to see my health like those bleached relics I found on the beach. Dried up, a bit of a lost cause.

If bones could be reclaimed as alive with lifeblood, maybe my own health could too. Maybe I didn't have to live inside a single story of what my diagnosis meant. The realization ignited a different understanding of what inhabiting a body might mean. Not the end of illness, but a different, more creative way to connect to the world.

Practice

CONNECTING WITH BONE

When I began sharing embodied writing with others, I often brought this theme of bones as a resource into our somatic explorations. Once, in a light-filled barn that had been remodeled with wood floors and large windows looking out to the forest, we practiced standing back to back with a partner and leaning back to feel a sense of connection and support through structure and bone. Slowly, I watched the group settle into the exercise, and the feeling of receiving support while simultaneously offering support to their partner.

"Wait!" cried one participant, halfway through. "Why can't I always feel like this?!" Making real contact with embodied support can change everything. In this practice, we play with bones as a portal to accessing new, bodied awareness.

Engage the Body

Lightly placing your fingertips on your opposite wrist, pause for a moment and simply feel. Then, inviting deeper bone contact, apply a little more pressure so that your finger bones meet your wrist bones. Do you notice any difference in this quality of contact? How does the rest of your body respond? Feel free to explore contact with other bones, perhaps bringing fingertips to kneecaps, clavicles, ankles.

Write

Listening from this place of contact, notice what your bones feel, say, hear, carry, or ask. Then, inspired by the title of Stephanie Foo's evocative memoir, follow the prompt: *What My Bones Know* . . . See what happens if you keep writing even after you feel you're done.

Deepen

Widening your attention, see if you can think of (or observe) structures that feel supportive and alive, rather than brittle and unyielding. Letting yourself be loose and full of permission, sketch one of these structures in your notebook.

FIRST PERSON

Trusting Support

Susan Lebel Young is a retired psychotherapist, author, teacher, and creator. She's also one of the most vivacious workshop participants (and people) I've met.

I plop onto a stone bench overlooking Casco Bay, sitz bones heavy. My breath deepens as I let my weight drop with the pull of gravity. I face the marina where my dad, an oral surgeon, had a sailboat he named the *Cuspid* ("because it cuts through"). His sturdy body and muscular arms rowed the dinghy, the *Bicuspid*, to the bigger boat. I land, open to sensation and notice. The tightness turns to jitters. The energy in my mid-body travels behind my eyes. Tears come. I note that the drips and wetness are both pleasant and unpleasant. I learned to hold such paradox with Johanna. I both welcome and deny the sadness.

Thanks to embodied writing I ask, "How do I trust that I am supported?" I let the tears run. At the same time, I feel the support of bone, like the mandible supports our cuspids and bicuspids, like the marrow, the stuff, the essence of the sea supports boats. I breathe and recall Johanna's words of arrival in our classes. "I acknowledge this land, the Wabanaki Confederacy, and reverence for our divine amazing bodies." I write it in caps.

Bones and marrow, common prompts in our embodied writing groups, escort my mind back to Dad. I write:

> *"His last few days, my arms held this now skin-and-bones man who let me be the strong one. As I buoyed his skeletal frame, he said, "Thank you, Sue, I couldn't have gotten out of the car without you."*

"I remember many years before, working in his office, seeing bone for the first time. I held the retractor during surgery, keeping the patient's jaw wide open. Soft gums became evident first, then white solid bone, bloody. My body weakened, legs wobbled, eyes widened. I watched Dad's skilled fingers scalpel the tissue. 'You have to make a big enough cut,' he said, 'to give the surgical field a lot of space.'"

A lot of space. I think of this often. Johanna says love is space and space is love.

Today I return to one of my favorite spots and give myself love-space, space-love to do nothing but touch into bone and marrow, the core of life.

Dad died of a bone marrow disease, a medical illness. But his amazing soul-self health lives in the marrow of my bones. And thanks to embodied writing, I can acknowledge and trust that support. I can bow with reverence to my divine amazing body.

LOST IN TRANSLATION

I sometimes joke that my husband, Jon, is what we hoped America would be: He's committed to service and social justice, a literal Boy Scout and builder who works to make things better for everyone. He is preternaturally kind and a Southerner.

So it was a bit of a jolt when, visiting my family in Sweden, he asked a question that made the room go uncomfortably quiet.

We were in the kitchen, the breakfast table laden with coffee, fermented yogurt, toast with cheese and lingonberry jam. An old friend was visiting from Stockholm and Jon turned to her and asked, "So—how've you been?"

Oh dear. The room came to a halt. Our friend stuttered, choking coffee.

"How have I—what do you mean? *When*?"

How've you been?, as my mother and I tried to explain, isn't a question you can just toss off to a Swede. Among my Swedish friends and family, it takes time to earn the intimacy of this kind of knowing.

But what's really lost here is that *How've you been?* has no entry point. No specific, concrete invitation that allows for an opening. Without this, where do we even begin? You might recognize this dynamic if you have school-aged children. Ask, "How was your day?" and you'll likely hear very little beyond *fine*. But, "What happened in the soccer game at recess?" elicits an entire story.

When we're beginning to develop our practice, asking us to listen inwardly without offering real entry points is a bit like this generalized *How've you been?* We want landmarks and guideposts to show us the way. Over the next few practices, we'll be very direct with the body, exploring this terrain in its tactile aliveness. As we deepen our somatic creative capacities, building familiarity and tools, we can widen our explorations to include the senses, touch, space, pacing, and much more. Taken together, these practices help us access, understand, and reimagine the stories we're holding.

We are so many things, so many ways, deeply influenced by the people and timing and places around us. Asking *How've you been?* is a broad brush often met with a pat answer (the cheerful American *Just great! How about you?*) that blanches the color from this wide palette. Jon, being Jon, understood and adapted accordingly.

"Sorry," he said, "How are you this morning?"

Practice
HANDS

Pause for a moment and bring your awareness into your hands. Are they resting, doodling, holding the pages of a book? And how about what they're feeling? The texture of paper? The warmth of a teacup? We use our hands so often and for so much that we can miss their supreme capaciousness. They both *do* and *feel.*

If you've taken an anatomy and physiology class you've likely seen the illustration of the cortical homunculus, a little man (only recently have models of women been developed) drawn so that the areas of his body are proportionate to the number of his sensory nerves. Which means that his back and legs are tiny, while his lips and hands, richer in sensory nerves than most other areas of the body, are enormous. You can see this in practice: Trace one gentle finger along your palm and you'll feel even the slightest sensation. The hands aren't only sensitive; they're also strong. That very same hand can become a powerful vise if, say, the salsa lid is on too tight.

In this way, the hands are uniquely gifted vocalists in the chorus of the body's parts. *They have range.* Not only strength and sensitivity, but open and closed, tight and soft, giving and receiving. As we move into direct work with hands, part of our invitation is to keep our attention actually *in* our hands. Notice the textures beneath your fingers and the things you love to hold, maybe a warm stone, flower petal, beach sand. Notice what you love to touch or be touched by. What do your hands tell you? What do they know?

The hands invite us to move into a rich series of somatic inquiries that might include the following: What am I reaching for / what am I releasing? What am I opening or closing? How do I build, make manifest, and realize my dreams? What do I love to touch? What do I love to be touched by?

Engage the Body

See if you can locate a small, tennis-sized ball (a rolled-up pair of socks will do in a pinch). Then, begin by massaging the hands: Press into the palms, grasp and release each finger, bring in a bit of gentle traction at the knuckle joints.

Next, using your ball on a table surface, slowly roll it around the palms, pausing and leaning into spots that feel stuck.

To close, rub palms together quickly, generating heat, and rest them on your heart/chest. Pause for a moment in appreciation of your hands. Consider what you've chopped, stirred, stroked, petted, made, soothed, punched, scratched, braided, baked, swept, pushed, folded, torn, planted, broken, mended.

Write

I fill my hands with / I empty my hands of . . .

Deepen

Hands speak. Sometimes, as with sign language, they are the medium of communication itself. They can also illustrate and adorn spoken words. My husband, for example, choreographs entire scenes with his hands. Installs drywall. Draws skyscrapers in the air. A friend told me once he was three blocks away, at night, in the fog, when he recognized Jon's silhouette, his wild gesticulations giving him away. Today, notice the gestures around you, the ways hands express what isn't necessarily named.

Practice
SHOULDER SEASON

We shoulder a lot. Individual responsibilities, familial needs, old wounds, collective heartbreak. It's no wonder that over years of working with bodies, this is the joint I hear about most.

The shoulder is such a capable joint that it's almost as if, if you'll allow me a little poetic license here, it forgets it's part of a whole body. Which makes the shoulder a particularly potent lens for examining our habits of bearing, how we organize around responsibility, and where we lose contact with our own systems of support.

First, a bit of anatomy: The shoulder is uniquely mobile. No other joint comes close to this range of motion. We're talking adduction, abduction, flexion, extension, internal rotation, external rotation, 360 degree circumduction in the sagittal plane.

For comparison, your leg, nestled deep in the hip socket, can do some nifty extension and rotation below the waist. But nearly a full circle of movement? Not close.

The tradeoff for this capacity is vulnerability. All of that ability makes it quite susceptible to injury. Put simply, because it can do *so* much, it often does *too* much. Shoulder injuries, tweaks, and pulls are woefully common.

Though this is less anatomy than physics, it's important to mention that the shoulder *exists in gravity*. I don't mean this facetiously. When we focus our attention solely on the shoulder, we're often picturing a disembodied joint. We've zoomed in so closely that everything else disappears. Everything, it should be mentioned, that *actually holds the shoulder in place*. Do you see how we're asking this capable joint to function while forgetting that the rest of the body is also here to support it? As virtuosic as the shoulder is it does not exist alone.

Friends, breathe for a moment and widen the lens to see how the shoulder feels when it's located within a whole framework. In workshops, people often marvel at how different it feels to experience this area as *supported by* the rest of the body. To include feet, hips, spine. By locating the shoulder from the ground up, we step into a whole different arrangement around what carrying might look like.

Of course, we aren't just talking about muscles here; you might recognize—just an iota—this pattern of supporting the world with your capacity and forgetting that *there are places from which you also must draw*. Of forgetting gravity, we might say.

The shoulder reminds us that as capable as we are, we need support. And it asks us important questions:

- What are we shouldering?
- What are our habits of bearing?
- More generally, how do we organize around responsibility?
- How do we connect to support?

Today, see if you can create pauses that reinvite your shoulder into gravity, resting in the supportive structure of your whole body. You might imagine that a kind friend occasionally puts a hand on you, gently nudging you to drop your shoulders down.

Our body metaphors are rich sites for listening. If we go in tenderly and with curiosity, we can discover a new blueprint for moving. Not an idea or a checklist of what to do, but a felt experience of shouldering more lightly.

Engage the Body

Begin by locating your shoulder in the body, drawing your awareness from the ground up:

1. Press feet into ground, alternating left and right.
2. Move awareness into the legs, rocking sitz bones from side to side.
3. Bring articulation into the spine, flexing and extending forward and back, then tracing your attention up through the spine, from the sacrum

through the lumbar (low back), thoracic (mid-back), and cervical (neck) vertebrae.

4. Arriving at the shoulders, pause to roll and shrug a few times.

Write

Things I've carried . . .

Feel free to get literal, metaphoric, and experimental in your writing.

UNDERSTANDING THE WORD *BODY*

On a rainy morning in April, Roger joined one of our online workshops for the first time. An artist in his seventies with glasses and a kind face, he sat against a background of a painting in different shades of blue. "Oh," he said quietly when someone asked about it. "I made that some years ago."

Today we were exploring the shoulder as a portal to writing. I'd always been fascinated by this interesting and singular joint, one that is anatomically hypermobile but also vulnerable and prone to injury. As a verb, *shouldering* speaks to carrying—our backpacks, burdens, and responsibilities. Taken together, the shoulder gets at the heart of a series of questions I wanted to explore with this group: What are our habits of shouldering? If we can pause to notice how and what we take on as a matter of habit, we might also explore what *supported* shouldering could feel like. As I moved through the introduction, I could see Roger taking notes, his mind whirring. He asked a thoughtful question to make sense of the work, but I knew that *making sense* could loop us into a cerebral approach that would lose the body. I tried to keep my answers short and turned toward movement.

We began from the ground up. First, pawing feet into the floor, left to right, catlike, then, rocking left and right, feeling the back of the legs, the hips. We drew our attention upward, through sacrum and spine, until we landed at our shoulders, now tapped into a whole structure of support beneath them. These simple steps disrupted old postural patterns and connected our awareness to a coherent whole. Then, we paused, grabbed notebooks and wrote into: *Things I have carried.* Ten minutes.

As everyone shared their writing afterward, we marveled at the unintentional collective *things carried* poem we'd created: my babies, my absence of babies, my mother's body, my worry, feathers, a secret, tapestries. There's often an echo in the images that come through; how is it that multiple people mentioned hay fields, bowls, hair, and grandmothers? We could never orchestrate this synchronicity, but it arrives even so.

It was after this first prompt that Roger turned to the group, a baffled expression on his face.

"How is this happening?" he asked. "Somehow I'm trusting my voice in this space. I'm *hearing* my voice."

Roger paused, seemed to catch himself. "Wait—is that the body speaking? Maybe I'm just understanding that word, *body*, for the first time."

Sometimes embodiment can arrive like this, catching us by surprise and upending our old definitions. As you explore these practices, you might notice how your own notion of body changes or shifts. Could the body be a way of knowing? A home? A friend?

Practice

HEART OPENER

"Why are you knocking at every other door? Go, knock at the door of your own heart."

—*Rumi*

Pause, just for a moment, and drop your awareness into your heart. You can even place a hand here as you bathe in this magnificent, electric, energetic center of you.

If we are sensitive beings, we know heartache. No wonder we're often overwhelmed or distraction-seeking. But let us also acknowledge that our sorrow is accurate; grief and suffering are part of what it means to be feeling, wakeful humans. As are celebration and joy. Our work has never been to solve or fix or estrange ourselves from our hurt. Our work is to occupy our bodies, to listen to the maps of our own pleasure and knowing, and to be able to take refuge not in leaving but in arriving more fully in the present moment, a place large enough to hold our sorrow and joy. As we do so, we build our capacity to care for ourselves and each other. Over these last chapters we've been exploring how we touch, carry, and build our way through our lives. We have, in many ways, been weaving a tapestry of capacious support for our heart.

Engage the Body

A heart-opening stretch can look so many ways. You could roll up a towel and lay back along the length of your spine or crosswise, so that the roll is parallel to your shoulders, letting your arms rest off to the sides. You might put your legs up the wall and simply breathe. You might fold yourself over a pillow (or willing pet!) and let your heart feel close. A sincere invitation to feel into a movement that lets your heart feel supported and at rest.

Write

Moving from this opening of your heart to the page, how might you acknowledge and appreciate this abiding space? Consider how it has endured, stretched, grown, grieved, celebrated. Follow the prompt *To you, my heart . . .*

PART III

The Stories We Carry

Bearing witness, taking inventory.

In part III, we'll widen our lens to consider how we became who we are. We'll take honest inventory. What are the feelings and stories we're carrying? The beginnings and endings? This approach gives us important maps for knowing, witnessing, and ultimately freeing up how we inhabit ourselves.

A PIECE OF BROCCOLI FLOATING IN THE UNIVERSE / ORIGIN STORIES

***When did your symptoms** start? Denote below the procedures, hospitalizations, and surgeries you've had.*

Most chronic conditions don't arrive all at once. In my case, there were a series of incidents and symptoms. None by itself an emergency but gradually increasing to a volume I couldn't ignore. Charting the beginning is complicated.

In the US medical system, documentation is a central component of health care. Every appointment begins with an intake form on which you're asked to chronicle your health record, including any allergies, symptoms, surgeries, hospitalizations, specialist visits, and medications. You do this on repeat. Which, if you're someone who frequents the medical system, can create a kind of intake fatigue as you account again and again for what's wrong.

Sometimes when I face these intake forms, I wonder what would happen if the questions were posed more directly and I could answer with lyric creativity.

Catalog below all the ways in which you are aberrant, how much, and for how long.

The first time I heard the word *colitis* was in a fortune teller's shop on Fourteenth Street in Manhattan. I was twenty-two and had handed over five dollars as a kind of joke, a dare to myself. The neon sign of a giant palm cast an eerie glow across the room. The unsmiling clairvoyant wore a yellow T-shirt and a steady, tired gaze. But then it got strange.

"Look, you have colitis. It's all over you! It's a disaster."

What? What was she even talking about? I had expected news on my love life, stories I could laugh about later. That night I asked a friend what colitis was. Something digestive, we decided. An old-fashioned disease.

How long shall we say you've had this? Always? Never?

Maybe the disease started nowhere I can detect at all. I could draw a picture of me, an infant on a fire escape in a snowstorm, napping outside. My mother, so freshly arrived from Sweden that her *J* went sideways at the beginnings of English words, turning *jokes* into *yolks*, held the strong conviction that kids need fresh air. An arrow to my colon, the caption: *The disease lies in wait.*

Stories have to start somewhere. But what do we remember? And where do we begin? I sometimes joke that before we were born, we were just a tiny piece of broccoli, floating in the universe. Perhaps we were. And while we do not have to know or even understand our origins, exploring them does help us see the ground we're standing on, the broccoli we rode in on.

When you engage embodied writing to chart your history, your memories get to leave the one-dimensional chronology of the intake form and include gestures, habits, fantasies, and the rich field of felt sense. Getting into your body allows you to uncover whole genealogies of posture. I remember once looking at a line of my sisters and mother seated on a bench, all of us, right leg crossed over left, left foot turned inward. Our bodies speak back to our origins. Not only the way we sit, but how we hold our fork, tilt our head to listen. One of my teachers used to say that we're all perfectly adapted to a place we don't live anymore. We learned to walk, move, and breathe in an environment of early childhood—a place we no longer live. Something as subtle as the way you hold a glass has roots; you learned how to do this in a particular place and time.

Feeling for our origins through our body is different than recounting our histories or analyzing our past. Those are fruitful practices, but here we're less interested in the linear story than getting loose and curious about what makes you *you*. We can free-range through our histories, getting expansive in the telling. I'm made of the matzo brei my dad cooked on weekends, the songs my uncles sang on the veranda, salty acrid air of the harbor. I'm made of learning to drive in Boston, paternal instructions that included, "Don't use your turn signals, Jo, or the enemy will know your plans." I'm made of tears. Of diagnoses. Of mystery.

The past is always reconstituted in the present. When we cast our net into the stories of our beginnings, listening creatively, we are also playing with the arc of our unfolding life, creating new futures, remembering that *this is not the only moment*. Perhaps we might think of ourselves as elders in training, finding ways to tell stories that foster a connection to those who come after us. Which, for me, feels like a richer, more bodied, more possible, and more inclusive way forward. It's an approach that offers a lighter touch to our unfolding lives, imbuing even an intake form with a bit of mischief.

And it might open a whole new series of questions: What are you made of? What beliefs and foods and places wend their way into the fabric of your making? What kind of broccoli (or river stone, cloud formation, land mass) were you once?

Practice

OUTTAKES OF AN INTAKE

One evening, when Nora was about three, she walked into our bedroom with a pen, a notebook, and a very serious look on her face.

"Mama," she said. "I have some questions for you." Thus began my favorite intake of all time. She could not yet write, but with each answer she scribbled a new line.

"Do you like to go to bed at night or hang out in the kitchen?"

"Um, I—"

"Is your face dotty? Do you want oatmeal? Does your lip budgeon out?"

"I don't know what 'budgeon' means." Nora turned to her paper, murmuring, "Doesn't know budgeon."

"Are your hands green?"

"No," I said. "I don't think so."

"Are you a turgeon or a pen?"

"What's a turgeon?"

"It's not a pen," said my child.

"Well, I'm not a pen . . ." More scribbling as I heard Nora say quietly, "Mama is a turgeon . . ."

How much richer our histories would look if our intake forms borrowed some of this flair for the absurd! In that spirit, our first stop in considering the stories we carry begins with a hat tip to my kiddo, making space for play.

Engage the Body

Invite yourself to get comfortable, making any microadjustments that help your body and mind know they can be easy.

Write

Grab your notebook and pen and feel free to compose your own wild questions. What inquiries would a bizarro intake form include? I can imagine a few . . .

- What is magic? How do you know?
- Assisted by your inner three-year-old, describe your current state using nonsense words.
- Hum the sound of a sunset. Now a sunrise.
- Apples or blueberries? Discuss.
- Do you like to stay up late or hang out in the kitchen?

Practice

FEET / I COME FROM

"People usually consider walking on water or in thin air a miracle. But I think the real miracle is not to walk either on water or in thin air, but to walk on earth."

—*Thich Nhat Hanh,* The Miracle of Mindfulness: An Introduction to the Practice of Meditation

If you are someone who walks, your feet are the only part of you that is in regular, direct contact with the ground. When we step into more conscious awareness of our feet, we also open new pathways of experiencing gravity, support, and balance. Physically and metaphorically our feet connect us with our roots and to what nourishes us from before and below.

Which babies, those geniuses, already know. Spend time with an infant human and you'll see them grasping, playing, and sometimes eating their feet. They're showing us how we might relate to our roots: playfully and with curiosity. This loose approach helps us wake up from places where we've been stuck, suggesting new ways of standing and walking in our lives. Offering ourselves space and attention and, yes, silliness, nudges us into present time, and brings lightness to our investigation of our origins.

Engage the Body

Choose any of the following feet exercises that speak to you:

- **Wake up:** Walk barefoot with your attention under your feet. Kick your heels up. Lie on your back with your feet to the sun. Place your feet in a warm bath of water.
- **Stretch:** Flex and point your toes; roll your ankles clockwise and counterclockwise.

- **Press:** Stand on a tennis-sized ball or a rolled-up towel to press into your arches, heel, and toe mound, lingering in spots that appreciate this attention.
- **Gentle traction**: If you're able to grasp your foot, begin by cradling one of your feet, using one hand to anchor the heel, while the other holds at the base of the toes. As you make conscious contact with the bones, gently pull your hands apart in longitudinal traction (along the length of the foot).

After you've worked both feet, come to standing (you can also do this from sitting or lying down) and bring your attention into your newly mobilized feet. Feel your roots extending downward and your crown extending upward.

Write

I come from . . .

Feel free to get very creative and free form.

Deepen

What might happen if you got very infantile with your feet as you consider questions like *What is my ground? What am I planted in? How do I connect to where I'm from and where I'm going?*

BLOOD DRAWINGS

One late October afternoon I stood in my friends' kitchen in Philadelphia trying to show them the house that Jon and I hoped to build. Nerdy and Megan are friends whose summer visits we look forward to all year long, people with whom we can share hilarious stories as easily as tender ones. Those kinds of friends.

"Wait, wait," I said, looking around for paper. "Let me draw it for you." Nerdy handed me a pen, and I stared into the middle distance. I wanted to show these dear and close friends the plans we had to build a house, a place we hoped they'd visit and would feel like home. Okay, I thought, screwing my face up in deep concentration. *The roof has a triangular pitch, and there are two windows on the second floor. A door over to the right.*

"Like this," I slid the paper over. We looked down at what I'd drawn. A long pause.

Reader, the house that a four-year-old might draw, a box with a triangle on top? That had more detail. We laughed until we cried.

But we never actually built that house.

In November, my disease spiraled out of control, COVID arrived soon after, and building prices skyrocketed. Along with the house, the whole notion of drawing or creativity was stripped away. "Draw" rehomed itself in the medical world, where I knew it best.

The word *draw* has its origins in Old Norse *draga:* to pull or drag, which is maybe why it has so many applications. Draw a bath. Draw a crowd. Draw the line. But in my experience, mostly this: draw blood.

IVs, infusions, blood draws. I have been poked hundreds of times across dozens of offices, hospitals, windowless rooms, beds, chairs. In my arm, wrist, the cleft of an elbow, and once—from a nurse who tripped over her too-long scrubs—accidentally into a nerve.

"I could do this blindfolded!" said one phlebotomist, making a joke as though to cover his eyes, my arm the donkey, the needle a pin. I forced a thin smile.

When I was in labor, I asked the nurse if she could please reset the IV higher up so that I could use my wrist. She looked at me curiously.

"Who asks to be poked again, while having contractions, no less?"

"Not my first rodeo," I exhaled between bracing. "Might as well do it up right."

But not everyone in my world shared that association. When Nora was three she handed me a picture she'd made, a great armless T. rex with sharp teeth, spindly legs, and a belly button, the most perfect thing I'd ever seen. Later she drew cartoons and graphic novels. Mini books. Murals on huge paper. As she entered middle school, her drawings got more elaborate. She spent hours shading, detailing, seeing. Developed techniques of texture and dimension that gave her images contour and shine. These were marvels of beauty and precision. *How'd she learn to do that? And what drove her to try?* One day I asked her.

"Honey, why do you draw?"

"It's relaxing," she said simply.

I had always assumed there were people who could draw (Nora) and those who could not (me). It had never occurred to me that drawing, a thing I had no talent for, could be relaxing. I judged myself as soon as I picked up a marker. Funny, since I had so much experience helping other people get looser and easier with their words. When it came to writing, I was determined to toss any outside idea of talent and reclaim the joyful, gentle practice of mixing body awareness and writing. This whole book, you might say, is an exercise in just that. Why did I imagine drawing was different?

And then I stumbled upon artist Wendy MacNaughton's Substack, *DrawTogether*. Her daily drawing prompts and laid-back support were so full of permission that they made drawing fun and approachable. "No rules in art!" she wrote. "You do you!" The more I drew, the looser I felt in my body. The more I noticed the world. I felt sudden affection for the curve of our dog's belly and the discarded onion skin on the cutting board. It wasn't called embodied drawing, but I recognized this way of engaging creativity that stayed loose in the body, noticing, being direct. Suddenly, I took joy in being an absolute beginner.

Sometimes the idea of tracing your origins or telling your story can feel weighted, like it requires casting back into your life to bear witness to the heavy and important things that happened. Engaging loose, easy drawing turns our attention to what is right here in front of us, creating its own kind of autobiography. Because the *way* we see, the things we find interesting or beautiful, says a lot about who we are. We don't have to explain why we find the handle of that mug so compelling; it just is. I mean, look at that curve and color, the way it catches the light. We've turned on our curiosity, inhabiting ourselves with new spaciousness. These marks on the page are a different way of bearing witness, of reclaiming what we want to draw into present time, where life is actually unfolding.

Practice

"DRAWING IS LOOKING AND LOOKING IS LOVING"

One of my favorite of Wendy MacNaughton's sayings is, "Drawing is looking and looking is loving." In this practice, we're holding MacNaughton's words close.

Engage the Body

Let your eyes fall on something nearby. Perhaps something you find interesting or beautiful. Then spend five or ten minutes drawing, staying loose and easy in your body and on the page. See if you begin to feel some affection for whatever object falls under the spell of your attention. Linger there, not worrying at all about technique or accuracy. No one has to see what you're drawing.

Write

When the drawing feels finished-ish, see if it might spill into writing. Maybe the object itself inspires you, or a memory of drawing, or a particular gesture leads you somewhere. Write where you're led.

Practice
SMELL MEMORY

When people first hear about embodied writing they often assume we simply mean sense-based writing. "Oh!" Someone will say, "So you emphasize taste, touch, smell, hearing, and seeing in the writing?"

The senses certainly are one way we gather information, and they can be a wonderful place to begin. But get in close, and the category itself gets shifty. Sure, there are the five major senses we learned about early on, but new categories of perception are added all the time. Interoception, proprioception, neuroception, kinesthesia, synesthesia. At one embodied writing workshop, when participants brainstormed senses they stretched the category even further: Timing. Velocity. Soul sensing. Intuition. Belonging. Love. Imaginal sense. Empathy. Tingle-at-the-back-of-neck sense. There are so many ways that the body knows and locates itself in the world.

All that said, the senses do offer us a rich and familiar way into writing with our bodies. But only one sense, smell, has a direct line to memory. Sound, touch, taste, and sight get processed through the thalamus, the kind of switchboard of the brain, for interpretation. *Oh, what am I looking at here? Is that the sound of dripping water?* Smell travels to the amygdala and hippocampus, key structures in emotional processing and memory. *Ew. Rotten. Do not eat! That waft—suddenly I'm in an alleyway in 1984 looking at a dead rat . . .*

After my grandmother died, someone handed me a small Ziploc bag containing one of her relics, a small pendant with stones forming a blue jay on one side, a cardinal on the other. Only months later, finally opening the bag, did I discover that the real treasure inside was molecules of her perfume, perfectly preserved. The sudden sharpness of her absence leveled me. In that olfactory signature were her soft hands, ice in a scotch glass at 5 p.m. sharp, the lilt of the way she said my name, distinctively Bronx Jewish. I would never feel—feel, in my ears and on my skin—the presence of this woman again. But suddenly, I could write it.

Smell can bring us to specific memories, to a moment. You've likely had the experience of walking somewhere when a stray waft of something hits you, instantly transporting you to a place or moment in your timeline. In this next practice, we're wandering the corridors of scent to explore the unique gifts of this evocative sense.

Engage the Body

If your nasal passages are clear, spend a few minutes practicing alternate nostril breathing: Gently use a thumb to cover your right nostril as you inhale through your left to a count of five. Then use your pinky and ring finger to gently close off your left nostril, remove your thumb, and exhale through your right nostril. Inhale again through your right nostril, close off the right and open the left nostril, and repeat.

Write

After a few rounds pause for a moment to bring to mind a scent from your life. Be willing to be surprised! Write into that smell, seeing where it takes you, what you notice in the scene, what details or feelings become available.

A note that when we're working with memory, we stay tender with ourselves, slow. If you notice that this exploration causes bracing or tightening, please take a moment to step away, recruit extreme gentleness, and reorient to what is here, perhaps revisiting some of our earlier work on connecting to resource.

FULL OF MYSELF / FEELING MYSELF

Let us consider two photos that show the arc of an entire story.

In the first there is me at five years old, owning the dance floor at my uncle's wedding. Arms flailing, hips rocking, red patent leather shoes doing . . . something with the beat. This girl is getting *down*, lost in the music and the raw delight of a dancing body. In the second photograph, me at twelve. It's 1990, so I'm wearing pegged jeans, a fuchsia mock turtleneck, and a Swatch watch. Hair covers half my face, and my arm braces against a large oak, like I can't quite stand on my own. I'm also sporting a look that suggests I'd like to disappear into the forest floor.

What happened in the space between these photos is such a remarkably common story, particularly for folks that are assigned female at birth (AFAB). As I approached high school, I tamped down my exuberance and started practicing smallness. I stopped swinging my arms wildly and snort-laughing. Less a conscious choice than a creeping posture: head down, shoulders stooped, face hidden behind a curtain of hair. Instead of the pure joy of *being* a body, I became preoccupied with the gaze that evaluated my body from the outside. Writer Melissa Febos describes this beautifully:

> Sometimes I think about going back. I imagine reversing the film of my personhood, reeling the spool to find the single frame where it all changes. As though there would be one murky celluloid square in which my body was taken away from me. Not just my body, but all the pleasures that came through it . . . the perfect freedom of caring about only what my body could do and never how it was seen.[5]

How it was seen became the primary organizing force of my body. I performed impressive contortions to avoid that most terrible of stamps, that I was too much. Or worse, that I was *full of myself.*

How I wish I could wrap my arms around my own young shoulders and dispel this myth, this determined diminishment. But part of getting older is realizing that our old beliefs were also our younger self's security blanket, what kept us safe. Ripping it away—banishing the habit—would simply communicate all over again that certain parts were unacceptable. So instead, maybe younger me would come along for a wander through the garden.

Because nature sure does love fullness. To walk through the garden in late summer is to see what this actually means: sunflowers pointing their heads to the sun, milkweed leaves thick with caterpillars, peaches so heavy and sweet that the branches snap under the weight. *Look at me,* they say, *I am feeling myself. I am so full of me.* Perhaps this secret message would be transmitted: To live fully, you'll need to fill up with what you are. With what you love. The music that speaks to you, the people who really see you, your foibles and fascinations, birthmarks, and scars. We do not have to pretend smallness to become acceptable, we might simply embrace what we already are.

And not only what we are individually. We can extend outward, recognizing fullness when we encounter it. Recently, on a light-up dance floor in a kitschy club, I looked up to take in the scene: a bachelorette party in Revolutionary War garb, high socks, and white wigs shaking it to Salt-N-Pepa's *Let's Talk About Sex,* a man in a plaid shirt and sunglasses moonwalking off to the side, my friends and me twirling and singing. All of us feeling ourselves.

As we take inventory, we also get to time-travel. To reverse the film of our younger selves to see what we carried, to offer what we know now. We get to bear witness to our old arrangements, noticing the intelligence that organized us in the ways it did, even if the cost was high. And we get to hold our own hands, wandering together to discover what living fully means to us now.

Practice

THE BELLY

Consider the metaphors we use with our soft middles: The belly of the beast, fire in the belly, to go belly-up. Supreme potency resides here. And yet when we speak of bellies we often relate to them from the *outside*. How they look rather than what they feel or sense. Which means that our belly—that seat of our knowing and intuition, our gut feelings, our second brain—is often hidden, tucked away, or pulled in.

Besides being a home for our intuitive gut feelings, this is an area of digesting, taking in, sorting through, letting go. A place where the outside literally travels through the inside. Which means the belly is quite direct in teaching us about nourishment in the largest sense, not just what food feels good, but what company, places, and experiences fortify us. Today you might ingest something that nourishes you or your belly-deep knowing. It might be literal food, a quiet moment, a canceled plan. Listen for what loosens the belly, what drops the shoulders, what settles you inside. *That* kind of nourishment.

As you sit with your belly today, your inquiries might include: What nourishes me? What am I still digesting? How do I inhabit or inhibit my intuition? What do I hide or diminish? What can I loosen; what can I let hang out?

Engage the Body

Begin by bringing awareness into your hands, imagining you can fill them with kindness, appreciation, and permission. Let them be infused by this feeling until they are so saturated they might simply radiate this feeling with easy generosity. Then, gently rest your hands on your belly. As you do, imagine them *filling you with supreme* kindness. Let this be a spacious meeting, making small adjustments as needed.

If you'd like to take this into movement, begin a gentle belly massage: Move your hands in slow rotation down the left side of your belly, across the lower quadrant, up the right side and back toward the left. You might echo this movement on the back body, using one hand to circulate the belly while the other parallels the circle on the back. Repeat a few times and return to stillness.

Write

When I am full of myself . . .

Deepen

Taking inspiration from Febos, imagine you could reverse the tape of your life to an earlier time when you felt less than full. Perhaps you made yourself smaller or diminished your own light.

Rather than give advice to this younger version of yourself, imagine what companionship or kindness you might offer them. Something they might truly savor. A field trip. A nap under a tree. A spoon of honey. See if you can offer them one of these joys that—surprise!—you yourself might enjoy today.

ORIGINS OF ILLNESS

Evening, so that the apartment windows reflected back the interior: dark reds of the late '70s, black-and-white television, an IKEA table of soft pine, record albums arranged on shelves.

I sat on the edge of the couch, but my legs didn't move. Couldn't move.

Get up, they said. *It's time for bed, the babysitter's gone home. C'mon.*

But my legs wouldn't do what I told them, and I was glued there to the corner of the gray couch.

I cannot remember how it happened, if in some small unconscious way my skeleton protested. Maybe it thought, *The baby, she's always being carried. The baby's coddled and carried. She doesn't seem to have to do anything.* My legs flopped, did nothing.

In the yellow light of the ER, the doctors checked my vital signs, administered blood tests, and handed me a cup of ginger ale, fresh and cold. After one sip, I swung my legs over the side of the bed and stood up, baffling everyone.

Years later, my father had no memory of the night at all, but my mother did.

"Yes," she said, "that's right. Your legs just stopped working. It was strange."

So strange. First, because a small seed planted somewhere quiet and dark, of miracles. What if all this—twenty years of this disease—could be gone with a cup of ginger ale? Hope sometimes being a brittle thing, a limiting thing, a blaming thing.

My father asked, with what I know he meant as kindness, "Jo, why do you think you're still sick?" It was a question he hoped could dislodge the pea from under the mattress, so everything might settle right again.

I wish I knew why I was still sick. Send me back to 1981, where all I need is a moment alone with my parents and a sugary drink to overcome my own paralysis.

Please don't tell, even as I am explaining patiently, again, that there is no miracle cure, I am still, always, secretly hoping for one.

Practice

A TIME WHEN I WAS SICK AS A CHILD

Remembering our first encounters with illness can help us see some of our original blueprints around health. How do we learn what pain means? What did it mean to be sick? These first memories of care (or absence of care) lay a foundation we live inside of during future experiences of not being well. Seeing them clearly can help us see the expectations we carry into encounters of illness, offering both appreciation for what was received and opportunities to meet our needs differently.

Engage the Body

Letting yourself get still and quiet, travel back to an early memory of feeling unwell. Bringing real tenderness to your hurting parts, what are you learning about what it means to be sick or in pain? What objects, people, remedies, or other details join the scene?

Write

Describe an early memory of being sick . . .

Session Portrait

FINDING NEW FRAMES

***In my one-on-one** sessions with clients, we often listen for somatic frames that help folks inhabit their bodies with more ease. In this scene, we meet Loretta as she finds new ways of holding old imprints.*

"When I knew I was in trouble, I hid," Loretta said plaintively. "It wasn't obvious; it seemed, probably, like I was still there. My brothers didn't notice. My mother was too deep into her cancer treatment. Some part of me," her eyes drifted to the left, "was gone. Which actually, when I got locked up, was a pretty good skill to have."

I'd worked with Loretta long enough to appreciate the beats she took in the telling, the f-bombs, the sly smile. In the early days when I met her for craniosacral sessions, she was skittish. When she lay back on the table, her limbs vibrated with a holding tension that echoed in her experience of life. She was intimate with trauma and had spent time incarcerated. Now in her mid-thirties, she was aware of how the feeling of being trapped and monitored still echoed in her body even as she had built a deeply supported life. Though we worked online now, Loretta had become so skilled at listening from within that I often felt as if we were still in the same room.

Her cat had moved into the scene, covering the camera with thick black-and-white fur. Loretta picked her up gently and gave her whiskers a scratch.

"You know what feels good?" She looked up.

"What's that?" I said.

"Knowing that's out of my life. Like I can have this sweet and good life that isn't tweaked and compromised. It's actually—it's a really good life." She *had* built such a good life. Loretta was in a loving partnership and was anticipating a new promotion at work.

"This is my chance not to be poor," she said. "To move up, do okay." She paused. All of this goodness ran against some strong original programming. "Things don't usually go this well," she said.

I asked Loretta what this edge felt like.

She paused, closed her eyes.

"I feel like a spinning top. Like, I'm seeing it all rush past, but I can't move anywhere. I'm just going round and round. I *like* the movement, but not the spin."

Loretta was gifting us a glimpse into how this moment felt on the inside. We stayed with the feeling, getting curious, neither rushing to analyze it nor fix it away. We wondered together if there could be a more supportive frame for her body here, one in which she felt more agency in authoring her own story.

I asked Loretta if she could imagine any small shift or movement that would let her keep this momentum but feel less spun out.

She smiled. Dropped her shoulders. "Skiing!" she said. "When I went skiing as a kid, it was effort, but it was so fun. I loved the feeling of going fast down a mountain." She recognized a different kind of movement, just a few degrees off the spinning top, that changed the whole story.

LOUD AND PROUD

The kitchen air at my grandparent's summer house felt thick with butter and spices. My sisters and I sat transfixed, watching our uncle Claes-Göran kneading dough on the large wooden breadboard. His arms worked efficiently to roll out the sweet bullar pastry, then baste and spread and cover. I snuck a piece of raw pastry, fresh with cardamom and sugar, still warm from proofing beside the stove. "Nja!" He cried, batting my hand away. "And what is this?"

Of my mother's three brothers, Claes-Göran was the most stubborn and least patient, the one who refused to slow his pace or clean up his language in the presence of children. Of course we flocked to him, hanging on his stories and jokes. One summer my sister Julia kept a running tally of how often he swore. We liked to tell anyone who would listen that our uncle Claes-Göran was one of the world's leading experts on the *Titanic*. He writes books, we'd explain, and travels the world setting up exhibits and displaying artifacts. His apartment in Stockholm was like a museum of marine relics.

But we didn't know that tragedy was part of my uncle's story too. How his community was decimated by the AIDS crisis of the '80s and '90s. The friends and lovers he lost. Only in hindsight did I come to understand that his fascination with the *Titanic* and other maritime disasters might have something to do with having lived through a series of slow-moving catastrophes. What a triumph it was to survive. And if you did survive, why not really live?

My uncle was (and *is*) loud and proud, not hiding his passions or personality. In his percussive, determined way, he showed us a version of adulthood that claimed its fullness. He knew what he loved and was utterly disinterested in anything that called him away from what mattered: Maritime history. Solitaire. Saunas. Dirty jokes. Singing. Baking. His partner of thirty years. His disdain for niceness but embrace of actual care.

Practice

FIERCE WITH REALITY

Florida Scott Maxwell writes, "You need only claim the events of your life to make yourself yours. When you truly possess all you have been and done . . . you are fierce with reality."[6] In this practice, we are claiming the events of our lives, calling back parts of ourselves or chapters of our lives that have been exiled, shamed, or hidden. As always, we're doing so with great gentleness, only picking up the threads that we can manage without flooding our systems.

Engage the Body

Imagine you are benevolently taking in your whole timeline. All chapters, all parts. Places of delight, places of challenge. Then, considering Maxwell's quotation above, open your notebook and consider what it might feel like to be fierce with reality. Was there a time when you told a difficult truth? A moment when you chose not to hide or felt hiding was the best option?

Write

When I am fierce with reality . . .

A GEOGRAPHY OF BATHROOMS

2003. It began gradually, with a strange urgency that didn't resolve. I had to go to the bathroom all the time. *Excuse me,* I'd say in meetings, pushing my chair back. *I'll be right back,* I announced, while interviewing interns. I rushed to close the doors behind me, racing a clock that no one could see, but what came out of me was all wrong, nothing I recognized. I was here in North Carolina for a job that was far from the coast of Maine, where I lived, and far from Jon, the man with kind eyes and calloused hands who I had just fallen in love with. At first, I assumed it was the climate that made my body unravel. In Durham, worms crawled out to the sidewalk where they fried in the sun. Kudzu, creeper, and long-needled pine tumbled behind my office and along the highway. The chaos and heat secretly infiltrated my body; my insides began to break free and run rampant.

My life became a geography of bathrooms. I was in the bathroom, or I was looking for bathrooms, calculating how much distance separated me from toilets. I learned to hate bathrooms with keys that delayed my entry. I wasted gallons of water, running the faucet to drown out whatever sounds I made. Paradise was a bathroom with a loud fan in an empty house.

But it didn't matter where I was. Blood was a constant fact, explosive and unpredictable.

One day after work I made my way to a pharmacy tucked in the back of a giant Kroger in King's Plaza. I walked past a phalanx of registers, racks of gift cards, flowers, display cases of gleaming frosted cakes in pink and green. The cashier, a round man in gold-framed glasses and a lab coat, seemed to be waiting for me.

"Well hello there, ma'am!" He was enthusiastic. "And what can I help you with today?"

I gave him my name, and he retrieved from the back a grocery bag of prescriptions, then enumerated the contents inside. Asacol (not pronounced *ass-a-call* as I'd somewhat hoped), twelve a day; prednisone, forty milligrams. Next, a small box of silver-wrapped bullets, the suppositories. I was to insert these at night but also whenever possible, at least twice a day.

Two children were skipping around the bakery department, lilting laughter, brown hair and brown eyes. I glanced over at the floral stands. Were those Gerbera daisies? Were they real? Electric blue, screaming red. They seemed to be of another planet.

"Ma'am?" I turned back to the pharmacist, who was holding a small canister of foam, describing how to insert the nozzle and spray into my rectum. His clinical distance was impressive. This entire bag of pills and foam and suppositories were missiles guided for my colon. I wished we could do away with the pretense and snort with discomfort, like middle schoolers.

"Do you understand these drugs as they've been prescribed to you, ma'am?"

I did not.

"Yes," I said.

That ma'am again. I was twenty-six. I wondered if this much rectal medicine pushed me out of "miss" and into another phase of life altogether.

I was willing to try these medications because they were the first stop in inflammatory bowel disease. They had no major side effects, and actually, they had no real effects either.

The true laboratory of my hope hid behind the bathroom mirror, in the boxes and bottles that lined the shelves, spilled over onto the sink. Marshmallow root. Turmeric. Enzymes. A remedy containing molecules of dolphin's milk from a homeopath who asked me if I had shark dreams. Probiotics. Chinese herbs.

The experiments extended to the kitchen, where muffins made from frozen pumpkin sat beside homemade yogurt and glasses of aloe juice. Printouts from blood tests, stool tests, strange tests that ran pulses to my fingers to test for allergies. An article on experimental porcine whipworm treatments. I was determined to figure this out. *To crack the code*. This was the language we used, imagining that the right combination of something would break this open, free me up. And so I cooked the herbal formulas, took the supplements, chased every notion I read about in online forums. I tried everything with the desperation of one who felt she was living inside a Frialator. I tried to maintain the appearance of someone uninterrupted by pain.

Practice

GEOGRAPHY LESSONS

If you have endured the ceaseless search for a way out or through, you are likely intimate with the sense of burnout and exhaustion that can take over. How geographies can shrink. In this practice, we want to recognize our trying and also offer the solace of space and witness that can shift the frame when we can't see a way out of our current predicament.

Engage the Body

Bring to mind a time when you felt your world shrink. Perhaps you were ill or living through loss or rupture. It might be a conflict you had with someone this morning. Or a moment of feeling lost in a crowd. Once you've located a moment, widen the lens of this moment to notice the surroundings.

Draw/Write

Taking your notebook, draw a map of the rooms and places you were moving through during this time. The bathrooms. Kitchens. Sidewalks. Hospital. Restaurant. Feel free to be crude or detailed in the recalling. Then, remembering our work in part I on resource, draw or write a resource that you might offer yourself in this place where you've struggled. A kind word. Soft sheets. A cool cloth placed on your forehead. Let yourself time-travel to comfort yourself in these spaces.

Deepen

Notice how this practice feels as a bodied experience. What happens when you make room for sorrow and care simultaneously? Does the geography change? Do new spaces or places become available?

Practice

REPURPOSING

In early 2008 I lived between the bathroom and the couch in a worsening flare, barely managing to eat. My daily outfit, green sweatpants and a fraying, threadbare gray sweater, seemed like a perfect expression of the way I felt inside. I wore it all the time, and then I wore it when I went into the hospital and stayed for nearly a week.

As the months passed, and my health returned, I confess I felt oddly loyal to that sweater. We had been through so much together. It lived in the drawer under the bed for years, daring me to toss it.

Perhaps you have some of these in your closet: hoodies, T-shirts, barely held-together pants that violate every rule of decluttering and cleaning. You don't wear them; they aren't beautiful. They take up space as odd cotton-poly relics of a time or place you can't quite shake. Sometimes, this detritus isn't just textile or even stuff. Sometimes our old habits and beliefs are their own kind of clutter, crowding out new experiences and taking up space. Maybe we've always been the one who never seems to have it together, or the one who always does. Maybe we're totally sick of these old beliefs and habits, ready to not need or hurt or bend in the way we have. But then . . . they were so useful once. They did serve a purpose. Anyway, that's how it was and always will be. Into the drawers at the bottom of our consciousness they go.

Years later, thinking that I wanted to make something for friends and family, I stumbled on the idea of potholders. So practical and easy—who doesn't need one? Potholders protect our hands from burning but without some thick stuffing, they're just closed up pockets.

Which is when I remembered that sweater. There was something sublime in cutting it to pieces, in giving it a new job.

This got me thinking.

What might happen if you could repurpose those old habits and put them in the service of new choices? Maybe, for instance, we learned that to get by we needed to take care of everyone else. But now, we get to also be *recipients* of our own strong empathy and listening. Or worthiness. Or trust. This is a different kind of decluttering. Instead of rejecting our old habits, we offer them new purposes. We get to discover what our old patterns gift us when they're free to inhabit new spaces.

Engage the Body

Bad habits. Good habits. Habit might suggest a rut we're stuck in, a practice of support or commitment, or even a way of sitting. If we aren't judging habit, what might it show us?

Begin by noticing your own posture. With much softness, see if you can make a small, even imperceptible shift. Perhaps moving just your eyes or loosening your jaw. Letting your hand rest in a new place. Notice how these small shifts might help you see your habitual posture a little more clearly. Rest for a few breaths, noticing how it feels to be in this slightly altered position, just a few degrees off normal.

Then internally visit the landscapes of your own habits. Perhaps there are stories you often tell, grooved ways of being, practices of comfort. See if you can bring permission and kindness to your explorations.

Write

I have a habit of . . .

Please bring your kindest self to this exploration. Your writing might be a list, a story, an observation, or not even writing at all.

Deepen

Pick one of your habits from the list above and speak to it gently, like an understanding kindergarten teacher. Where else could this habit play in your life? What new areas could it explore?

Practice

AN AUTOBIOGRAPHY OF LOVE

I have fallen in love so many times.

The first person I had a terrible, aching crush on was a Swedish boy eight years older than me who wore rolled-up pants, played the soprano saxophone, and barely acknowledged me. He had a snaggletooth, bangs brushed to the side, and his name, to the delight of my friends back in the States, was Jerk. Never mind that it was pronounced *Yahrk*. "Oh," they chided, "Asshat was already taken?"

But maybe these humble beginnings set me up to find love in unusual places. Lovers yes, but also friends, places, plants, bodies of water, experiences, animals, excellent sandwiches, popcorn paired with a Negroni, the way my friend Meredith slurps her tea, how our red dog Rosie turns her giant chest to the sky when a potential belly scratcher enters the room, the sea smoke that rises over the ocean on exquisitely cold mornings.

Such a partial list. But an autobiography of what we've loved is a luscious way to reconstruct the past. This is a practice to deepen our work around developing resource that we began in part I. There are so many ways to connect to what feels good.

Write

See if you can get very loose and easy with yourself. Loving, even!

Write an incomplete list of what (and maybe who) you've loved . . .

Practice
TURNING POINTS

It was just a firefly. One lost, lone firefly that drifted through my Brooklyn window one hot summer evening, circled the room, and flew away. But it was a turning point in my life, a moment when I finally understood what I needed to do next in my own life: *Leave.*

Years later, I'd wonder why that small bug got my attention when I'd ignored all the obvious signs. I had felt so adult, moving to the city after college and finding a job and apartment. I worked at a nonprofit, where my desk was crammed in the corner of a back hallway. My bedroom window faced a brick wall in an apartment that was robbed, infested with roaches, leaked, and caught fire, twice. And the relationship I had moved to the city for was slowly and spectacularly falling apart. The trappings of adulthood felt more like traps, and I walked through my treeless neighborhood like a ghost. I wished for air and space and sun, but in the city these were commodities I couldn't afford.

Then came that firefly, igniting a sudden sense of wonder that burned off the cobwebs of all my excuses. I didn't know it at the time, but this was the spark that would set off a series of decisions that ultimately put my life on a different course altogether.

We can only chart turning points in hindsight. There isn't a before and after when you're just doing the next thing. But I did wake up a little. Soon after, I noticed a paragraph at the back of my elementary school newsletter mentioning this small bilingual school in Latin America. Six months and two interviews later, I moved to Costa Rica.

That first night in the rainforest, after the car had finally ascended the long dirt track, I stepped outside into the night and gaped. No cars or voices, sirens or people, but an unending cycle of riotous orchestration, chirps and buzzes, hums and creaks. Lightning lit up the valley below. Something glowed in the trees. The forest breathed. I did too.

A year went by. A year of teaching and living and laughing off the husk of a person I'd become. One night I sat in the dark outside a salsa dancing class and fell into conversation with a handsome visiting carpenter. I told him of my plans to move to Maine and attend a documentary school. "This one?" He asked, pulling out an old copy of the school's magazine, one he'd taken along because it contained an article on carpentry. He lived in the same small city. Twenty-three years later, we are still sharing plans and talking into the night, raising a child and garden and whole life together.

Sometimes the thing that sets us on a different course is barely perceptible. Other times, a flashing light (or lightning bug) grabs our attention. Perhaps larger shifts are only the accumulation of a million moves until one finally turns the tide. Thinking of life as an ongoing series of turning points helps me feel the nearness of possibility. Even this breath could be a moment when a different path opens up.

Engage the Body

Spend a minute simply breathing, getting curious about the transition from in-breath to out-breath. Then bring to mind one of your own turning points or transitions.

Write

The moment it changed . . .

What was the before? What was the after?

Session Portrait
CULTIVATING KINDNESS

***Sometimes we're so used** to our inner voice that we don't notice the way we talk to ourselves. In this scene, Agatha's astonished question, "Wait, you talk to yourself that way?" reveals a whole new way of embodying care.*

"Wait, are you serious? You want me to go take my probiotics NOW? During our session?"

I sighed. I truly didn't love telling Agatha what to do. As a longtime participant in my practice, I had come to adore her self-knowing and her saltiness, her defiant, absolute intolerance for facile pleasantries. I expected some pushback.

But today she felt defeated. We were meeting online, and though I couldn't see the piles of paper just off the screen, I knew she was struggling with not being able to do basic things. (Agatha would correct me here to say, "I cannot get shit done, and I'm sick of it.") She was wading through deep, ongoing disappointment with herself and her inability to follow through on tasks.

Agatha had practiced as a healthcare provider for decades, and the hallmark of her style and personality was a very direct approach to care that had endeared her to a large community of devoted patients. Which made her current state all the more painful. Despite being a health expert and deeply knowing what she needed, she could not summon the energy to do any of it. Neither getting something from the basement, nor mowing the lawn nor, as it turned out, taking a probiotic she needed to treat her dysbiosis—an imbalance in her gut. Which led us to our current moment.

"I am sick of all this self-care," she said. "I just can't get myself to do any of this." Agatha lived on her own and was sixty years old; she had a robust circle of friends and a beloved dog, but no one was making her do this. So I pushed, just a little.

"Yes, I'm serious. Take me with you, let's go into the kitchen and take care of this right now." She looked at me through the screen. Blinked. Paused. Her voice broke slightly.

"I don't know why that makes me tear up." A sigh. "Okay, let's go take care of this." I watched the scene behind her change as we moved through the house. Glimpses of her cabinets, her turquoise fridge, her dog Beauty in the background. I heard the water fill the glass, the spoon stirred the water. And then she drank it down.

"Good job, Agatha," I said.

"Ha!" She laughed. "Good job for a glass of water! I bet that's what you say to your daughter." I considered this. I'm sure I've said "good job" to Nora for things that are unremarkable, but I realized this was not that voice.

"Actually, that's what I say to *me*."

Agatha stopped, taking this in. "Wait—what? You talk to yourself this way? Like you say, 'good job' when you drink a glass of freaking water?" She was incredulous.

"I do. When I have to take my medicine, or go in for a blood draw, or get another IV, or give a stool sample, I am very kind to myself. I say, *Good job, sweetheart, we didn't love doing that, but now it's done.*"

"Really."

"Really."

"Okay, fine," she said. "That's sweet. But that's what you say *after* you've done the thing. How do you get yourself to do these things that are such a terrific pain in the ass? That you just cannot muster the energy to do?"

I considered the question. "I have to recruit some part of me that knows we just have to do this. I don't think of it as self-care, it's just basic care. Part of what I need to do to be here. But I have to acknowledge the resistance. So I say, *okay, sweetie, I know you really don't want to do this, but we are going to take care of it now. We just have to, so here we go.*"

Agatha looked at me. In fact, until she'd called me out, I don't think I'd acknowledged this to myself.

"How'd you learn to do that? Was it when you had a child?" It was such a good question. I felt the wide maw of time, how far I was from the barbed, chastising, and disappointed way I used to talk to myself. So many things happened in the gap between shaming myself for being sick and learning to live more peaceably with my limitations. Parenthood played a part but so did writing that incubated this kinder connection between my body and my self-talk.

“Maybe?” I said. “But I’d just rather be a friend to myself. It’s hard enough already to manage all this.”

Agatha shook her head, smiling.

“This is big,” she said.

“This is big,” I repeated. And then, because ribbing is our love language, I went on. “But it is absolutely not the first time we’ve talked about this! It’s just, you’re hearing it.” We guffawed together.

“I’m sure you’re right,” she smiled. “But I didn’t hear you till now.”

Practice

INNER FRIEND

The way we talk to ourselves matters, because . . . we can hear us. In this practice, we're trying on the feeling and language of being a kind friend to ourselves. In many ways, our journals are a home for this open-hearted, nonjudgmental space, but here we're taking it a little further, recruiting a part of ourselves that is both fierce and fiercely loving.

Engage the Body

Take a moment to bring your attention into the potent line of your spine. Feel this verticality extending deep into the heart of the earth and up through your crown into the sky. Feel it as a midline that is both supple and strong, organizing the whole field of the body.

If it's available, you might bring to mind a time when you felt fierce with your own knowing, perhaps in care or protection of yourself, a person, or an animal. Notice this alchemy of kindness and strength. How does it feel? What kind of voice does it have?

Write

Let this kind, knowing, center-of-your-spine voice tell you what it knows. *What does it have to say about the care you need? How does it want you to care for your deep health? What does it offer about living well from here?*

VOX HUMANA

"One of the dangers of technology today . . . is that we hear the human voice less and less. We hear the robotic imitation of it. So the sound of the human voice suddenly does something [snaps fingers]. Vox humana *to me is what it's all about."*

—Studs Terkel[7]

A year into teaching middle schoolers, I realized that if I really wanted to help my students write and engage with the world, I needed to go back to school myself. And so, thinking that real-life observation and reporting skills might help, I enrolled in the writing track at the Salt Institute for Documentary Studies. But a few weeks into the program, it was clear my aim had been off. The good stuff was down the hall, in the radio room.

Unlike traditional radio newscasts, documentary radio mixes voices with narration and sound to tell a compelling story. While we writers labored over our words, moving them, lifeless, around the monitor, the radio students hefted their tape recorders (still tape back in 2002) and microphones out into the world to interview and gather sound. They were having so much fun down there. They created storyboards and wrote narration so engrossing you felt like you were hearing stories around a campfire. I would find myself pushing my chair farther and farther back from the table of writers to eavesdrop on the radio instructor's lessons. It finally dawned on me that radio might actually be a *better* tool for helping young people write and get out in the world. By year's end, I had enrolled in the radio training and started hefting a microphone of my own.

I didn't know it at the time, but the beginnings of embodied writing were there in that small move down the hall. Because part of what drew me to radio was how much more *bodied* it felt. We went out into the field to gather recordings, holding our mics near a stranger's mouth, our voices reverberating in conversation. We wrote, but we cared deeply about how the words sounded, not just what they conveyed. Even now, as I type this, I'm speaking out loud (thankfully, out of earshot of my family) because I need to feel how it resonates. Does the language land with a recognizable truth? Or am I in my head, explaining but not really present? Radio began to show me how to recognize when a voice came from a whole self.

Over the next decade, I taught audio storytelling to teens in Durham, North Carolina, to young people incarcerated in juvenile detention centers in Maine and eventually around the country, as the director of a national youth radio network for young producers through a platform called Generation PRX, at the Public Radio Exchange (PRX). It turned out that radio *was* a perfect tool for working with young people. They loved the power that a mic offered, disarming even the most rigid authority figures. They loved that the medium was visual but not image-based. And amid all the posturing of teenagehood, radio was an oasis of authenticity that matched their absolutely precise bullshit detectors. They knew immediately if they heard a truth glossed over or a rule that made no sense. They called people on it, often to their faces. My students were brave with their questions, candid with their answers, and unflinching in their observations. Again, and again, these young producers showed me the essential importance of voice and being heard. And that if we are supported to do so, we can powerfully retell the story of our unfolding lives. As a group, we celebrated when someone's voice came from the beating pulse of their own discovery. When language felt direct and true.

Teaching writing through radio gifted me an unexpected recovery from my own stiff schooling. After decades of thinking that writing was laborious and cerebral, radio demanded I loosen up. Writing for broadcast isn't literature; it's less sophisticated but more direct, demanding that we use language that is fresh, clear, intimate, and honest. We told our students to *let go of the flourishes and say it true. Stay loose; imagine you're speaking to someone who knows how funny and great you are.* Radio only works if you sound like you, not an impression of who you think you're supposed to be. Your voice, your singular, bodied voice, is one of the great gifts you have to offer the world. Why broadcast any voice but your own?

Years later, when I left public radio and began to practice as a bodyworker, I'd discover how these two apparently opposite worlds both hinged on a capacity to listen to what is actually being communicated. Whether we're working with the tissues in a body or the nuances of our own writing, we need to drop the script and pay attention with our whole selves, listening for the spark beneath the surface. Doing so is the difference between going through the motions and showing up with meaningful presence.

Embodied writing would gather all these strands together, but it all turned on that first tug toward voice, body, and the conviction that our stories are ours to tell. Here in our embodied writing practice, we're perhaps beginning to develop a bit more courage in knowing and naming what is true for us in an embodied way. Maybe you've had moments when you surprised even yourself by articulating something you hadn't known until the words spilled out, reverberating with a truth felt within. Naming matters. When we begin to speak from our whole selves, we change the trajectory of our unfolding lives.

Practice

THROAT AND VOICE

"We often tell our students, 'The future's in your hands.' But I think the future is actually in your mouth. You have to articulate the world you want to live in, first."

—*Ocean Vuong,* On Being[8]

The throat and neck house that most important instrument: your voice. This is a rich portal for singing and speaking, naming and knowing, harmony, resonance, dissonance. Like the hips and pelvis, this area is a kind of channel between above and below, a meeting place between thinking and feeling. A place where we speak our visions out loud.

Like writing, the voice can be a place to practice permission, to get out of your head and let your creations and your discoveries unfold together. Sometimes using your voice isn't only about sound at all but the silence that lets it all breathe.

Engage the Body

The throat, neck, and voice are integrally connected to shoulders, head, diaphragm, chest and—of course—heart. Across this area is the platysma, a great flat muscle that extends from your chin, over your neck, and down to your clavicles. This is the muscle that pops out when you extend your lower jaw with exaggeration.

Anchor your platysma by placing both palms on one side of your upper chest and pressing into the tissue, then extend your head backward and side bend away from your hands until you feel a stretch in the front of your neck. Repeat on the opposite side.

Spend a few moments appreciating this area that speaks, sings, sighs, and vocalizes. Can you imagine a future of possibility in your mouth, as Vuong names above?

Write

My voice . . .

Deepen

Today, try getting very playful with your voice: Sing along with the radio, talk to your plants, surprise yourself with your own silences and noises. From this wide, expansive place, consider some of these questions:

- What is my language?
- Where does my voice flow? Where does it catch?
- How does my creativity find expression?
- What is my relationship to speaking? How is my body part of my speaking?

PART IV

Naming. Grieving. Celebrating.

Developing range.

With tools in hand for listening from a nervous system, understanding our origins, and attending to present time, we turn to honest naming of our experiences even when (especially when) our bodies and lives no longer follow the script of our plans. We'll explore moments of coming undone, learning to listen to our body as a friend, and writing as a way to understand and inhabit our body from within. As we make space for grief and celebration, we widen our range and capacity.

DEVELOPING RANGE

In the big room at the top of the stairs, we sat amid a small explosion of rubber balls in various sizes and colors. They bounced around the cushions and rolled across the floor, creating a kind of joyful chaos. If you had walked in just then you might have thought this was a gym class or a nascent ball pit rather than an embodied writing workshop. Which, considering our meeting place, it could have been.

On any given night, the Good Medicine Collective in Portland, Maine, was host to dance parties, readings, movement classes, acupuncture clinics, and healing circles. Often when I walked in there was the smell of just-burned palo santo and candle wax. Other times, the distinct musk of human effort, the boxing bag in the corner still swinging on its hook. Its cathedral ceilings and wood floors looked out on the wide expanse of the Casco Bay Bridge and its endless whoosh of traffic, making the space feel like a hovering still point above the harbor's activities. Years before this building became a center for health and transformation, it was a bar called the Ice House, with the tail of a small plane sticking out from the roof, a distinctive feature of the Portland skyline. Which is maybe why I thought of it as a place for landing and arriving. For diving in headlong and seeing what happens.

On this evening, we were using these bouncing rubber balls to dive into the fascia, the continuous membrane of connective tissue that wraps each nerve, muscle, organ, and bone in your body. The system is such an interconnected network that learning to read the fascia is a little like discovering a secret treasure map of how the body organizes itself. A single point can reveal where the tissue glides easily and where it's dense or adhered. I've palpated clients' ankles and felt an immediate tug from their jaw or shoulder or hip. And when I'm facilitating workshops, fascia is a powerful teacher in how to inhabit a body with greater ease.

First we chose our tools. There was a brief scramble as each person selected their rubber balls. Kate chose pink, Marissa the thicker, pearlescent one. Lara opted for a small yellow ball, pebbled, like a basketball. I invited the group to simply notice, from sitting, how they felt in their chests and shoulders. These before pictures can help us notice later shifts.

"Fine," said Ranya. "Maybe a little pulled down?"

"Concrete! Quiet concrete," said Lara.

"Constant low-grade tension," offered Bea.

"Good!" I said. "The fascia is a doorway to working with the whole body, and our experience will be unique to our own body. We want to pay attention to how we name what we're feeling."

"When it comes to the fascia, healthy tissue is supple and yielding, rather than tough and condensed."

"Imagine if the world was like that!" Someone cut in. "What if we had this approach to strength—yielding, soft, and stretchy instead of forceful and dominating?" There were nods all around. Someone suggested an overthrow of patriarchy and a new fascial world order. I went on.

"Unlike the mind, which would like to plan and predict the future irrespective of the body's experience, the fascia responds to stimuli in present time. When we listen from the fascia we receive very direct feedback from the body about *what feels better*. And what feels better works better. There is no committee, no book, no text thread, no weighing of options. We simply and slowly move towards yes. *Move a little to the left, there, there. Yes.*"

I heard someone let out an exhale of recognition.

"The fascia wants to move in opposing directions. Laterally, vertically, it loves the feeling of stretch. Literally and figuratively, it's helping us build the capacity to trust in a wider range. But here's the kicker: *It stretches more in response to time than pressure*." I paused to make sure the group understood the significance of this approach. In most other areas of life, we're taught that effort will get us there. But in order to shift, fascial tissue needs you to wait until the body softens in a deeper unwinding. Like the nervous system, meaningful change happens in abiding presence, not willful pushing. In craniosacral work, we call this way of working without an agenda *listening to the intelligence of the field*. When it's ready, the body can show new possibilities that our minds couldn't imagine.

"Okay! Let's try this out."

Each of us lay face down on the mat, a ball compressed between sternum and floor. With each breath, we softened into gravity, noticing places that felt taut and tight, slowly shifting so that the ball moved along the clavicle and into the shoulder girdle. As the group settled in, I felt the room go internal and quiet, entering a more meditative space in which each person was in conversation with their own tissue.

Afterward, we paused to touch in again with sensation. I heard folks exhale into the stillness. Eyes closed.

"My breath feels so available," said Lara. "And my back is closer to the ground."

"My chest feels more open and breathable."

"I didn't realize I was making any effort before, but now I'm aware that things feel easier. I can't explain it. Things are changed from here."

Poetry lands differently when we feel this easier inhabitation of our bodies. In the stillness, I shared Danusha Lameris's "Let Rain Be Rain," a spare, gorgeous poem that invites the reader to be direct with the living world. I offered the group a prompt. The scratch of pen on paper filled the room.

Transitioning directly from the stretch of the fascial body to the stretch of our mind fortifies the instinct that every part of us has *to move.* It's as true for our bodies as it is for our writing: Stuck places have limited movement. In the tissue, when muscle fibers adhere they have less freedom and more pain. (Most of us are familiar with the discomfort of a knot.) Stories aren't dissimilar. We listen for the organic propulsion of freshness and surprise as well as the sag of pattern and overwrought thinking.

When we make generous room for our bodies to stretch in opposite directions through the fascia we're widening the range of our stories too. All of which helps us build our capacity to meet the moment and companion each other through all of it, building a collective trust in the greater swings that carry us in and out of balance, like the breath, like the tides.

So far we've been developing tools for listening to a nervous system, taking inventory, and understanding our origins. In part IV, we're making space, stretching wider and deeper and following the call of the fascial system to move toward *what feels better.* Not by strategizing, bypassing, or locking in a plan, but through flexibility and trust. It's a little like rolling out an inner welcome mat to signal: Be easy here.

Practice

BREATHING OUT / BREATHING IN

Like the two wings of a bird, exhalation and inhalation are inextricably linked together. In this practice, we explore both sides, building range.

Exhalation

Exhalation sends the breath outward, drawing the belly in. It's both a letting go and a calling inward that creates an opening for the next breath. It's also a reminder of the essential need for pause. Like a rest in music, or what singers call a luftpause, these spaces turn noise into song.

Physiologically, the out-breath is also a more direct route to greater calm (what's also called down regulation). As James Nestor, author of *Breath*, explains, if you're feeling stress, the easiest way to calm yourself through breathing is to exhale more than you're inhaling.

In this culture that often tells us to scale bigger and go further at every opportunity, exhalation can get a little lost. But this gathering-in is fundamental, it reminds us that emptying and filling are equally necessary.

Engage the Body

Bring to mind a place or time in which you easily exhaled, relaxed, or turned inward. Then rest your attention on your exhalations for a few rounds of breath.

Write

I gather and let go . . .

Practice

INHALATION

Of course, letting go is twinned with beginning again. In our embodied writing workshops we often explore inhalation as a spring movement: waking up, igniting. Walk into a room where something delicious is cooking and notice how your breath organically moves to bring this scent inward. With inhalation, the belly fills, the aroma arrives, we start something. We become porous.

Rather than asking us to join life elsewhere, inhalation invites the world to join us *right here*. It suggests a fullness that's available in each moment. In that spirit, we'll move to really open our breathing.

Engage the Body

A few options below to help open the area around the lungs:

- Either from a seated position or in tabletop, with hands and knees on the floor, practice cat/cow: On an inhale, drop the belly toward the floor and look upward, extending chest and head. On an exhale, round the spine toward the sky and tuck the head toward the chest. Repeat for several breaths.
- Using a small ball (tennis, massage, or bouncy), position yourself with your back to the wall, and place the ball between your shoulder blade and spine. Gently bend and straighten your knees so the ball tracks along the edge of the shoulder blade. Repeat on each side.
- You can continue to explore stretching tissue using the small ball, applying pressure along the underside of the clavicles and across the pectoral muscles or on the side body beneath the armpit and into the upper ribs.

Afterward take a few breaths to notice this newly opened space.

Write

I fill myself with . . .

NOT ACTUAL PAIN

Dusk looked purple outside the doctor's office in Harvard Square. I had walked the short distance from my graduate school classes to the student clinic with my eyes cast downward, trying not to activate another spasm of debilitating pain. Sitting under the fluorescent lights beside a long Formica desk, I felt pulled downward by an invisible chain wrapped around my intestines. I stayed in this awkward angle, bent toward the rug with eyes raised up, as if in supplication. I kept my breath low and shallow.

This doctor was a stout man with a shock of dark hair whose voice was brittle and exasperated. Later that spring, I'd catch a glimpse of him driving a cherry-red convertible through Harvard Square and feel momentarily stunned by this vastly different persona.

"Johanna," he said, "if you're flaring as much as you say you are, I urge you to take the medications I'm recommending." We had had this conversation before.

I felt threadbare. I conceded that I was in a good deal of pain.

"Well," he said, "there are no pain receptors in the colon, so you can't really be in pain. You might have some referred pain, but not actual pain."

I inhaled slowly. My *not actual pain* had nothing to say to this.

A few months later, the doctor administered a sigmoidoscopy without anesthesia. The test was designed to examine the colon from within by way of a camera inserted through the rectum. In my memory, the room goes flat and white, nothing but a cold table, the monitor, and a long, black rubber tube. Was the tube an inch wide? A mile? It traveled up my colon by degrees, the doctor releasing a valve of air, inflating my insides like a tire, pushing the instrument further and further until my body was a zeppelin, floating away.

Hovering above the room, I looked down to see myself, tempestuous and yowling, curled on the table like a question mark. The doctor's eyebrows arched, face implacable. Rising skyward, I saw myself as a preteen, climbing the steps of the Harvard Coop to look at posters and flirt with boys, and over here, the ribbon of the Charles River, and my six-year-old self riding in the backseat along Storrow Drive, calling out colors on the building domes as ice cream flavors. Red, blue, and gold. And finally I could see across the harbor and beyond the ocean, and there was my grandmother, picking black currants off their branches, and my own toddler body running naked across the lawn.

Even from here I could make out the noises that came from the office below; my voice crying out in a pain I'd detached from. Pleading noises. I thought how odd and stripping this process was, to be both dehumanized—hooked to probing machines that whirred and clicked—and so animal: wild-eyed, crying, curled in the fetal position.

The doctor wiped his brow. Said something about this normally being a painless procedure. I must be extremely sensitive. I felt the twin shudders of shame and confusion. Was there a choice? Was the pain I felt *not* pain? I wasn't sure how to orient to this body if what it signaled was deemed unreal.

On the way home, I tried to stitch the pieces back together. What had happened in there? The doctor didn't recognize my pain as real, rendering me illegible to the health system I depended on. I knew this experience was less an outlier than confirmation of depressing statistics. Mounting data confirm what most women know: Our pain is taken less seriously, our wait times for treatment are longer, and we're more likely to have our pain misdiagnosed as a mental health issue.[9] For women of color and folks who are marginalized in any way, all of this maltreatment magnifies.[10] Which presents patients with a terrible quandary: How do we find appropriate care when what we report about our experience is so often dismissed?

Unknowingly, I had been indoctrinated into the secret society of medical performance: At the moment of greatest vulnerability, we perform the delicate two-step of displaying competency while demonstrating a restrained version of allowable pain. All designed to convince our caregivers that we are reliable narrators, worthy of believing. A dance both exhausting and heartbreaking. If you know the steps, I am sorry.

Over decades in the medical system I've encountered a wide range of practitioners and approaches, and not all of them required this dance. Years later, when I visited a different clinic about some new pain, the nurse offered me a radical bit of repair. She paused, put down her clipboard, and turned to me with her full attention. "Why don't you tell me what you're afraid of," she said. "Maybe then I can help and reassure you."

That was all I needed. Permission to be human and to be seen. Her gaze didn't break through my tearful list of worries, and her kind listening got me to the truth of my own predicament, less terrifying when it was named.

What might happen if we could let go of monitoring our reception and believability and attend to what our pain was showing us? This more direct approach would help us know its various expressions so that we could discern the difference between white hot emergency pain, lower registers that ebb on their own, and the many, many flavors in between. As patients, familiarity with our symptoms is an area in which we have a good deal of expertise. Practitioners who acknowledge this truth have a far greater chance of meeting us where we are. It's an inclusion that is itself a kind of healing.

Practice

WHAT MY PAIN KNOWS

Essayist Sonya Huber writes, "I wish my pain made me beautiful . . . Instead it is just pain, wordless and desperate for expression."[11] In this practice, we're attending to that desperation, offering our pain space to express itself.

Engage the Body

Take a few breaths and locate an area of discomfort in life. This might be physical or emotional, a past heartache or a pressing worry. Remembering our work in part I, call in your skills for holding space without scrutiny. As you consider this pain, notice what areas of the body light up, what sensations, textures, and colors you feel.

With compassion, invite this pain to express itself on the page. As you do, a gentle reminder to avoid leaping into fixing, counseling, or figuring out what this all means. Simply offer free-range expression.

Write

What my pain knows . . .

Deepen

Many of us who've lived with illness or loss have been on the receiving end of well-intentioned suggestions that make us, just speaking personally here, slightly insane. In another essay, Huber shares this gem: "I have tried and I enjoy yoga. But if you tell me to try yoga, then I will have to fight you. You will win, but I might nip at your jugular with my sharp incisors first."[12] With humor at your side, explore some of the good, bad, or ridiculous advice you've received over the years. How might you take this even further? What might you say in response?

NONCOMPLIANT

February 2008. A room high up in the hospital. Whirrs and clicks, beeps and chirps, the measurement of life is audible but spare. Each time I was admitted to the hospital, the stay was a bit longer, but this time I didn't trust that I'd leave.

Jon sat by my bed, watched the IV drip, tried to make me more comfortable, which was not possible. "Please," I told him, "don't tell anyone I'm in here." I texted my closest friends, emailed work to say I was out of commission, but otherwise I held my hospitalization like a gross, quiet secret. What language could I even use to describe what was happening? All of this—the disease, its symptoms, my inability to get better—felt humiliating, like it finally put the lie to any pretense of competency. I wanted nothing. To fall to the bottom of the ravine and wait there in the dark alone.

The doctor visited me daily, trailing a small cadre of interns, a movable pool of clipboards and white coats. He checked the notes on my chart and again suggested surgery or stronger medicine, options I resisted with what I had left. His exasperation was plain. I was one of *those* patients. I asked too many questions; I was convinced there must be other options. My chart likely contained that medical catchall, "noncompliance," a shorthand for "not doing as instructed." Another area where medical language lays bare the thinking beneath it. Patients can have a million reasons for not following instructions. If they're unhoused or underresourced, if their home isn't a safe place. If alcohol or drug addiction makes care unfeasible. If, like me, their own wishes and beliefs are giving them pause.

Early on in my illness, a friend said that we should name my colon and suggested Helen, after Helen of Troy, she who sank a thousand ships. So was it destiny or cruelty that the woman on the other side of the curtain from me was a patient named Helen, whose responses were limited to the single word, *WHAT*.

"Helen," the nurses said, "I'm here to check your vitals."

"WHAT?"

"I'm here to check your vitals!"

"WHAT?"

"I'M HERE TO CHECK YOUR VITALS."

"WHAT?"

Pause. "Helen, all set, you did great."

"WHAT?"

"YOU DID GREAT."

This conversation, one thousand times. Except at night, when she cried out in her sleep, "I'D LIKE TO BUY A VOWEL!"

One night I found myself wandering the hallways at 3 a.m., pushing my IV alongside me. I stared out the windows at gray frosted roofs, helicopters, startled to catch the reflection of my own sticklike figure. What had I become? My mouth tasted of metal, and I could not remember what all this effort was for. I had tried for so long to deny the truth of my body, and in here I was *only* a body, one constituted of drugs and delusion. Skin and bone and bowel, Delaudid, prednisone, antibiotic.

Jon brought me news of home, salves, food, and a gift my friend Sepideh had sent, a book of poetry and photographs from a Zen monk called *Making Love with Light*. The doctor, on his next round, aped at the title, yukking it up to his audience: "Well what are you reading here?" He chortled, showing the book around. "Well, oh well—this kind of material might be contraband!" Guffaws all round, knowing looks.

The next day the doctor reappeared on his own. He announced, his voice a rope of irritation, that the choice was mine: I could take the medication he recommended, or I could find myself a new doctor.

I decided to do both. New doctor *and* new medication.

Sometimes healing comes not so much from a breakthrough as from no longer having the wherewithal to do it the same old way. I couldn't keep chasing the appearance of fine. I wasn't fine. I needed help, which included medication and, as it turned out, a new doctor. I needed a truer accounting of my condition, and to lean into, rather than away from, the people who cared. I didn't want to sleepwalk through life, buying vowels at 3 a.m., insisting on a reality that didn't exist.

Practice

TRUTH-TELLING

Hearing outsiders—particularly those in positions of authority—diminish, dismiss, or otherwise disrespect us can be a deeply overwhelming experience, one marked by both grief and anger. In this practice, we're offering ourselves the solace and potency of heart-centered language that tells the truth about what we feel and know.

Engage the Body

To begin, breathe. Remember gravity, perhaps letting your body feel heavy and supported. Roll your eyes and tongue. Bend your spine forward and back and side to side, in horizontal planes. Invite yourself to get a little loose: Might it feel good to roll your shoulders, press your feet into the floor, or take a long, audible sigh?

Then see if you can create a line of awareness from your heart to your brain and then out through your eyes. Could you play with letting your looking be directed by curiosity, even love? Turn your head slowly, side to side, feeling this out.

From here, two options:

- Position yourself in front of a mirror, offering yourself this heart-centered gaze. What resonant language recognizes your true self? How might you express kindness with both levity and depth? What accuracy of character and experience?
- Simply letting your eyes be guided by your heart, where do they settle? What new beauty do they recognize?

Write

Bring to mind an encounter with a description of you or your circumstances that felt reductionist or judging (language that could be coming from the inside . . .). Pause. Create some space to notice how the words land, even recruiting some of your own humor to notice how bananas inaccurate this description is. Then call in the practice above to meet the moment with kinder and more resonant language, like a friend, cheering you on.

What I really want to say . . .

Deepen

Explore writing from this heart-centered gaze. What will you see when you let your heart lead? When you let solace inform the exploration?

DREAMING IN THE SHAPE OF OUR ACTUAL BODIES

A month after an ER visit for another complication with her chronic illness, a friend was talking to me about her ambitious plans for an upcoming project. She knew, she said, that her body would pay a price for this exertion, but the thought of *not* doing it felt just as bad.

"Because what am I supposed to do? Just . . . accept that my body can't do what I want and lie around? Just throw up my hands and give up?"

I know this voice. At different moments, I have asked *exactly* this exasperated question. For a good part of my twenties and thirties, I felt like I was pushing with all my might against a door I desperately wanted to open. On the other side: a life that followed my plans. One I imagined as easier, free of disease or at least its symptoms. So close—if I could only figure out how to get through. In the meantime, I kept making and canceling plans, projects, whole careers.

But if living with a chronic illness has shown me anything, it's that my aspirations are not separate from the truth of my condition. All those plans you made? You can't do *any* of that. Even if you don't live with limitations, you know there are simply times when, as the Quakers say, way closes, and the path we thought we were following disappears. This can take us to some gnarly places.

Our culture abandons broken things. Capitalism understands relationships as transactional; it elides ability and value. So when we can't *do*, this gets to the very heart of our self-worth. And because all of this feels so painful, it's hard to untangle the belief that, in not-getting-well-yet, *we've* done something wrong.

When we push ourselves into shapes we cannot make, we leave our body *and its knowing* behind. When we only listen to the part that wishes this all away, we are wishing ourselves away. And can I just say—with woefully too much experience here—that living like this is exhausting?

It's difficult to hear what your body is telling you when you're holding tight to a vision of how you thought this all would go. And there are absolutely times when obligations (financial, familial, or otherwise) make the notion of "listening to your body" laughable.

But.

Our bodies keep demanding that we live into the stories they're *actually* telling. And sometimes, when we soften our plans around our true shapes, we can hear a soft sigh of relief beneath the ringing disappointment. Perhaps because, as terrible as it feels to drop the version of life you thought you were living, if your body cannot survive it, it is not the life for you.

Which can feel like defeat, especially given the metaphors we use around illness or trauma, where war is the common trope. We'll beat this cancer, we'll win the fight against Crohn's. But speaking personally, I'd rather live in a garden than a war zone, particularly when the battlefield is my body. I'd rather see what blooms in this particular landscape even if it's not hospitable to all things. Regarding my health this way moves me out of domination and into collaboration with my larger life. Maybe, like me, you are also interested in decolonizing your dreams. In understanding that you're not only out to conquer what lies before you but that the thing you're moving toward is also, in some ways, moving toward you.

Co-creation doesn't ask us to break ourselves in conquest; it includes pauses and rests, meals, distractions. It allows us to wander. This approach to ambition includes times when it really might appear to anyone looking like we're not doing anything. Because we *aren't* doing anything. These shape-shifting periods are not engaged with doing at all. We're listening somewhere else.

Nearing fifty, it feels like that door I was shoving my shoulder into all those years actually opens *inward*. When I let in what I actually am, I can sit in the beam of my true capacity and shape, which lets me navigate the dance of what I *plan* to do and what my body *can* do with a little more grace.

I don't have a neat solution for my friend, but I want to draw her close in solace and understanding. To wonder together what it might feel like to dream in the waking truth of our bodies.

Practice
SHAPE CLAIMING

In this practice, we make space for our grief and disappointment. We hold the twin pulls of frustration and acceptance; offering ourselves the grace of both/and to hold open the possibility of new pathways and consider what might be moving toward us even as we're moving away from a future we imagined or a path that was thwarted.

Whether you are faced with limitations of a body, a circumstance, or your old material cycling back again, you're in good company here.

Engage the Body

Take a few moments to connect to and move the hands, neck, and mouth.

- Gently palpate the hands, opening and closing the palms. Rest for a few moments with attention in the hands.
- Bring awareness to the neck, throat, and mouth. Play with gently rolling the neck, opening and closing the mouth, moving the tongue, and maybe a lion's breath (strong exhale with mouth open / tongue out / eyes wide) or three.

Write

I truly wanted . . .

Were there things you wanted to do or try? Aspirations that might have been possible? Lots of permission to explore frustration, hurt, or disappointment.

Then, after a pause, reread your words, allowing space to feel whatever they invoke. See if you might offer grace and kindness to the body that's carrying you through this.

Deepen

From here, taking in your true shape, see if you might feel into other possible futures. Perhaps you feel a gentle connection between you and this imagined space. What might you plant in the garden of your life? What seeds might thrive in your particular soil?

Session Portrait

FINDING YOUR TRUE PACE

Rejoining the world after *a difficult time can present its own complexities. In this session portrait, we meet Ian to explore the nuances of pacing.*

Ian had carved out a bit of space in a small room for our virtual session. Through the screen I could make out white walls, wood trim, and a large bureau off to the side. Like me, Ian lived with inflammatory bowel disease, and the last few times I'd seen him I'd recognized the gaunt, drawn features of a body living in unending flare. Ian and his partner had a small child, so alongside the ravages of his autoimmune disease were the demands and exhaustions of early parenting.

Today Ian seemed better. His new medication was working, and his face and body had a new fullness. He was starting to get used to leaving the house and had energy to do things again. But this new territory raised its own set of questions. When you've been braced to survive, spaces of reprieve can be deeply disorienting. What do we do with this new blush of energy? How do we find our boundaries when limited capacity isn't doing it for us?

When life reanimates after coming undone, we can't simply press play on the tape and pick up where we left off. Suleika Jaouad writes in *The Book of Alchemy* that when she was declared cancer free after four years of treatment, she found herself, "lost in transition, stuck between a haunted past and a future I couldn't yet imagine."[13] I shuddered with recognition when I read this. Perhaps you do too. In the early days, I'd come out of a Crohn's flare eager to do all the things I couldn't before, and then, overextended, I'd flame out, symptomatic, bathroom bound. I was a decade into the disease before it dawned on me that I wouldn't be going "back" to the way I'd done it. I'd have to figure out an entirely different way through.

Now here was Ian trying to navigate his way through this new world of feeling better, asking real questions about how to live life from here.

"What do you notice," I asked him, "when you feel into this experience of having energy again? Do you have a bodily sense of it on the inside?"

Ian closed his eyes and settled for a few breaths.

"I have this sensation in my limbs," he said. "A kind of manic rushing. It's like they're ready to fly into the activity of preflare, to grasp feeling useful and capable again. At the same time," Ian sighed. "I have this bone-deep exhaustion. Like even the thought of getting started is laughable."

This was such a precise description, one I recognized. I asked Ian if he'd ever driven a manual car.

"Yes," he said with some obvious bafflement. "I drive a Bronco." I knew it was odd to bring up auto transmissions in the middle of a discussion about healing, and that vehicle-as-body metaphors can feel like a tiresome trope when you're living with illness. Still, I'd come to think of what Ian was describing as a very specific *missing-third-gear problem.*

Regardless of what (or if) you drive, you might know the feeling too. At the center of the body, a sensation that is slow and condensed, *maybe* able to start, but barely able to go. First gear. At the extremities, everything spinning, and fast, a kind of rushing forward. This is fifth gear: all speed, no real power. Works for going down the highway at seventy but has no spark to get us going. Taken together, a kind of thin, surface-level speediness above a core of very little energy at all. As though ignition and momentum were strangers to each other.

Our engines don't work this way and neither do our bodies. We need transitions. We'd like third gear. Actually, we'd like to move between *all* the gears, to fluidly shift the pace for the moment, adjusting our inside capacities with outside needs.

But how do you find this elusive pace that's neither spinning nor stopped? Ian had taken the first step by naming and noticing the feeling. We talked about bringing extreme gentleness to this awareness, neither scrutinizing, blaming, nor demanding an explanation for *why* this had happened. Then, gathering the same tools we've been developing over these pages, we tried to slow down the experience to see what else might be available.

I asked Ian if he could describe what this meeting place between fast and slow felt like. Was it a sensation he could bring into awareness? And if so, could he discern any clues that would help us really see it?

"Well," he said, "I don't know if I feel it in my body, but—there's a brittle line there." He gestured in front of himself, paused. "Actually, it's softer than that. More like a membrane."

The more we let the body guide our inquiry, the wider this space became. Instead of two distinct speeds, Ian began to notice that there might be a conversation between the speedy part that needed to prove capacity and the part that sought to protect his body with stasis. He was still in discovery, but the frame shifted and felt easier to inhabit.

Practice

A TRUER PACE

In this practice, we'll explore our pace as it changes, moment by moment. We'll be staying loose. And if we get a little too serious, may I gift you the Swedish word for speed, which is—to my never-ending delight—*fart*. An exit is an *utfart*, a speedbump is a *farthinder*, a speed trap: *fartkontroll*. I am not making this up, and I am sharing it so you can remember to bring permission and play to this inquiry. To meet yourself not with a checklist of rules, but a wink and an encouraging smile.

Engage the Body

The poets are great teachers in imagining our way back toward a truer pacing that has flexibility and fidelity to life as it's being lived. Louise Erdrich's poem "Advice to Myself" and John O'Donohue's "Blessing for One Who Is Exhausted" each bring such gorgeous language to the notion of pacing that third gear suddenly seems like a very inelegant metaphor indeed! Both poets ask us to deal directly with the moment at hand. The body is primary. The dishes are not.

Bring to mind a time or place where you felt like you were operating at your true pace; a moment that felt good to you and perhaps had an absence of effort, rushing, or split. This might be an activity as simple as mowing the lawn or floating on your back in the water. Get curious about this feeling, maybe noticing a congruence between inside and outside.

Write

My true pace looks like . . .

Practice

A CONVERSATION BETWEEN GRIEF AND CELEBRATION

I once heard the poet David Whyte say that a good elegy is a conversation between grief and celebration.[14] Stretching our capacity means visiting this conversation, noticing how these apparent opposites are intimate with one another.

One of the great loves and losses of my life was Charlie, a giant of a dog in stature and soul. Though he passed away years ago, missing him is still raw. A collie-shepherd mix with a coat of faded brown, red, and beige, Charlie had ludicrously white legs, as though he had put on bleached knee-highs. He wasn't cuddly. He did not lick. If you tried to snuggle him while he lay, he would get up, irritated, shaking himself off. His preference was to lean his whole body into you, or to wait, just off to the side, working the perimeter. He was steady and constant and heartbreakingly gentle.

Charlie could fly in praise of love and the arrival of someone he was happy to see, a whirling blur, impossibly fast, leaping and sailing in circles around the cars. His whole body cried: *Yes! Yes! Here we are! Let us move!* And off he took, sometimes crashingly.

When we got him from a shelter up the coast, Charlie had been abandoned twice already. He was wild and skittish. At six months old, with big feet and a body that would soon double in size, he would whine and jump and throw himself. His movement was careening, without regard for objects or people (or their bad knees) that might be in the way.

But we stuck together, and in that abiding, he came home to himself. Grew into the gentle watching giant he was. He did the same for us; his touch and constancy melting us into who we were to begin with. All of us, irrevocably marked by love.

Engage the Body

Bring to mind something or someone that marked your life in a meaningful way. Let yourself linger in the details of what you notice, the feeling that suffuses your chest and hands. What are you celebrating? What are you grieving? Is it possible to let these parts coexist and know each other?

Write

What might a conversation between this grief and celebration sound like?

THIS IS IT

The sailing center my father ran on Boston Harbor had an impressive fleet of boats whose names reflected his love of astronomy, science fiction, and mythology. Driving the launch through the mooring area you'd pass *Amber*, *Yoda*, *Entropy*, *Mars*, *Warp Drive*. One season, two new Sonars were added to the fleet, and my dad told my sister Melina and me that we could each name a boat.

A poetic, wordy nine-year-old, I wanted to choose something beautiful and hopeful that would please the adults. I named my boat *Spring*. Melina, six years old, with dimples that lit her face when she smiled, turned to my dad.

"*This Is It*," she said.

"What—what is it?" my dad asked.

"The name of the boat: *This Is It*."

"Are you sure?"

She was. Capital letters were emblazoned on the stern: *THIS IS IT*. When people called to make boat reservations, we'd tell them, "Okay, you'll be taking *This Is It* at four o'clock."

"What is it?"

"The boat. *This Is It*."

It took me years to appreciate my sister's brilliance. When we don't dress up or oversell or rebrand or shine up what is actually here: THIS. This is it. Let it be simple, unadorned naming, a clear witness of what is here, whether awesome or awful.

Which is not how we often do it.

If you've experienced the loss of a loved one, or a diagnosis, or grief of some kind, you've almost certainly been met with the opposite of clear seeing. You may have heard some version of:

I'm sure it happened for a reason.

Just look on the bright side.

Well at least . . .

Even writing those words I feel the bracing that accompanies these well-intentioned denials. *Cheering up* is the opposite of acknowledgment; it's a secret communication that the pain we feel needs to go away. Not having your reality recognized can feel enormously lonely. Closed off from connection, we find ourselves unintentionally settling deeper into hurt and the conviction that we'll always feel this way.

In these moments, I like to call Melina's boat into memory, like a floating message on the horizon: *This is it.* It reminds me to return to the clear seeing that says yes to whatever is present. Sometimes the phrase takes different forms, like the inartful but true *This sucks, and I love you.* Or the wonderfully awkward *I don't know what to say right now, but I'm here.* Perhaps you also feel the difference in your body when you try these out, the smallest softening of effort. The words matter less than the honest showing up.

Practice

CLEAR SEEING

When we offer clear seeing that doesn't try to bright side the circumstances or offer platitudes we are practicing solidarity—sol—at its roots: whole, entire, undivided. We're saying: I'm with you through the full catastrophe. It's a companioning that opens the possibility of meaningful shifts, ones that unfold in their own right time.

Engage the Body

Begin by bringing your awareness into your field, noticing how your body, mood, sensation, or energetic capacity feels. Staying with this awareness, see if you might turn up the volume a bit, magnifying what you notice. Are there particular places in your body that feel held or tight, shoulders that lift, hands that grip? See if you can locate words that describe these feelings, letting them be fully evoked through metaphor, texture, image, posture. Do you feel like a swarm of bees? A redness? A flat stone? Lots of permission to make this expression neither nice, pretty, nor legible.

Then see what shifts when you invite permission into exactly what's here. Is there anything that happens—insight, awareness, settling—when you let these sensations simply belong and bring a quality of *this is it* to what you notice?

Returning to your body, turn your awareness to how you feel after bearing witness here. Better? Worse? Looser? Seen?

Write

Know that I am . . .

Practice

DIRECT OBSERVATION

When I was in graduate school, studying for a degree in arts in education, I had a wonderful professor, Steve Seidel, who taught us a technique for observing art or poetry with kids. The idea was not to interpret or judge but simply name what we saw. One by one we'd go round, and each person would name a single thing they noticed.

Looking at Matisse's *The Dance*, for example. *There are five people. The background is blue and green. I see a belly button.* As each person spoke, we'd have to look more closely so as not to repeat what had been named, which meant that new connections revealed themselves. *One knee is on the ground. Two hands are just barely touching. No eyes are visible.*

The more we looked, the more we saw, and the more our appreciation of the piece deepened. The process gifted us an important lesson: Our simple observations led to more meaningful connections than scholarly analysis or deciphering. Considered witness was its own kind of delight and discovery.

Engage the Body

If you can, find an old photograph of yourself. Spend some time purely looking. Treating this as an object of great art and composition, list all the things you simply see, without naming, judging, or interpreting. Challenge yourself to keep noticing, even after you think you've seen it all.

Write

What have you discovered in this image? What new connections have you made?

Session Portrait
TIMING

Sometimes, learning to reinhabit *our bodies can be accompanied by its own kind of reckoning as we face the question: Where have I been? Ali shows us one way of meeting this moment.*

"I wish it hadn't taken me this long," Ali said softly. A photograph of a bee pollinating a flower hung on the wall behind her, and she leaned forward, resting her hands in the lap of her overalls. Ali had gentle eyes and calloused hands and had just come in from a morning of planting.

"I just wasted so much of my time cowering, you know? Feeling like I had to apologize or make everything okay. This feels like my birth story all over again; I got abandoned, and then I abandoned myself."

We paused in the quiet. Ali was adopted as a baby, and she described needing to earn her belonging as a feeling she'd carried for most of her life. Now in her sixties, she felt like she was finally learning to inhabit herself. Trusting her voice. Feeling her own spine. I felt it too. Ali seemed more settled in herself and less preoccupied with managing other people's opinions.

But that awareness carried its own kind of grief. As she mourned for all that she had missed, Ali asked tender questions. *Where have I been? What took me so long to listen to myself? Why did I waste so much time?* I have heard some version of this question from folks who are twenty-five and forty-five and seventy-five. I myself have asked this.

We might begin by appreciating how brilliantly Ali constructed *a self that made it through.* Whatever compromises and adaptations she made helped her survive. We might also pause to acknowledge that our economic system does not exactly encourage inward listening. Capitalism may center the individual, but only insofar as that individual is an insatiable consumer. Self-care is taken to mean a spa day—a brief interruption from regular programming, not an *inhabited* individual vested in care for self, other, animal, and planet. It's a courageous step, to move off the constrictions of old programming and tend to a life that is more bodied, compassionate, and connected.

But what I really want to say to Ali is *I also wish it didn't take this long.* Healing happens on a mysterious timeline over which we have little control. Occasionally repair happens quickly, but more often it's the accumulation of small elements that have lined up to deliver us exactly here, supporting this precise change. It's an opaque set of factors that carry us, imperceptibly, from one reality to another.

Over time, Ali has developed more access to a sense of her inner little one, the small child who was abandoned and also adopted. I asked her if she had a sense of how this young version of herself felt about things taking so long. Ali put her hands to her chest and paused.

"Actually, she feels soft." A smile bloomed on her face. "She only cares that I'm here now."

Healing is an ongoing process. We know this if we live with a chronic condition. We know this if we're tender-hearted. We know this if we've plain survived. But I do sometimes wonder if the secret to healing is very much like the secret to a good joke . . . *timing.* Which means that if we're paying attention, there are also a thousand right-timed moments that might offer us a kinder way of meeting ourselves. Moments where we choose, against all odds and training, to be our own ally.

Practice

I AM NOT FOR EVERYONE

There is a wonderful punk rapper / art poet in Portland, Myles Bullen, who has a song called "iAmNotForEveryone." Sometimes, when I find myself wound around the axle of someone else's opinion, I call in the phrase.

I am not for everyone.

After a lifetime of monitoring other people's feelings, the phrase feels like a wild gift. An embrace of the radical practice of *not* pleasing.

What we wear, say, how we dress, these very words. *Not for everyone.*

Perhaps try that phrase in your mouth and body and see how it feels.

I am not for everyone.

Edgy? Liberating? Maybe a nudge toward noticing that insisting everyone be happy with us was, just the tiniest bit, a secret strategy we developed early to stave off abandonment? But if we are committing to a practice of permission, we need to grant everyone the sanctity of their own experience, which means returning outside opinions to their rightful owners. Also being accountable for our own. We may not be adaptable to all situations or pleasing to all people, but we can begin to discern what and whom we are *for.* It's a kind of devoted attention that will clarify what matters.

Write

Part of developing range means noticing when we have wandered into territory that is not for us. Being gentle and playful with yourself, make two lists: *What are you for? What are you definitely* not *for?*

AGAINST RESOLUTION AND RESILIENCE

My friend Megan's partner drowned on the cusp of his fortieth birthday. I remember the heat of that clear blue day, and Megan's taut voice through the phone. *Matt is gone. He's gone*, she said. Jon and I got in the car, driving past strip malls and gas stations to meet her at the river. I had the sudden awareness that sometimes things veer quietly off course and sometimes they cleave heinously, ripping a hole in the fabric of life.

In the days and months that followed, I saw how quickly the world wanted Megan to put her pain to use, to find the silver linings. Her bestselling and beautiful book, *It's OK That You're Not OK*, came out of the crucible of that time, as she learned firsthand how utterly terrible most of us are at accepting loss. She's become a fierce advocate for grievers around the world, helping them access support that understands, "Grief cannot be fixed. It can only be carried."

Megan and I were already friends—she's whip-smart, funny as hell, and a delight to be with—but we found new resonance in our different kinds of loss. Grander forces had wreaked havoc, and we both lived inside a life that wasn't the one we thought we were choosing. Also, neither of us were very good at following the script that demanded, implicitly or explicitly, that we turn our suffering into a story of resolution or resilience.

I know I am not alone in feeling the constraints of this script, which mostly demonstrates a supreme unwillingness to acknowledge what's here. So much space opens up when we don't demand our suffering make itself beautiful. Space we can inhabit. Space that puts making room for our experience ahead of making meaning of it. What might happen if we allowed the truth of what we're living inside of without requiring it to prove some sort of worthiness?

Creativity absolutely can be a deeply healing force, but I cringe a bit when creativity is treated like a cure or an antidote to suffering. Megan writes, "When we separate the creative process from a need to solve or fix things, it becomes an ally. It becomes a way to withstand grief, a way to reduce suffering, even if it can't change the pain."[15]

If we don't banish our suffering, creativity is a friend, calling us back, making the world more habitable and inclusive, wide enough and wild enough to hold the totality: the mysterious, the unresolved, the shadows, the beauty. Ironic, maybe, that when we don't ask our losses to resolve into stories of recovery or strength, they can show us the gold of a life willing to claim its fullness.

Practice

HEALING AND THE INNER COMPASS

There is a slippery and persistent question that lives under much of the work I do: What does healing even look like? Is it real? Do we know it when we see it? Even the word *heal* is a complex and evasive little bugger. We know we aren't working in the binary of broken and fixed, so does "getting better" mean . . . anything?

And then I meet a dog who has some answers.

It is at the last stop on our last day of camping that we meet her. With our dog Rosie bounding ahead, we take a trail that follows a small stream up through the woods to a waterfall that cascades into a deeper pool, the water dark with tannin from fallen pines. Coming down the trail are two men and a dog—a stout, gray Australian mix of something, with black spots on her back and a few across her nose. We stop to say hello as the dogs scamper and play, and then it's time to go.

"Smokey!" they call. "Smokey, come here girl!"

But what Smokey does is not come here at all. First, she trip-traps up the rocks and moss, crosses the brook, crosses again, and finds a place where someone has dropped crumbs. Then she gets distracted, tumbles and tussles with Rosie, crosses again, sniffs some ferns, and remembers those crumbs.

"Smokey!" They call again. And she does *look* at them this time, but walks down the hill, past her humans and straight into the cool black water. She plops down on her haunches in the middle of the pool with a look of deep satisfaction and extends her neck to admire the trees above.

I wish I had a photo of her at this moment to show you: cooling, entirely pleased. Imagine delight sitting in water, delight as a thick, gray black dog: There she is.

They are patient, her two human companions, gently saying her name until, eventually, she does amble over.

"How long have you had her?" we ask.

Five weeks, they say and explain that Smokey had spent her first year and a half of life chained outdoors in Oklahoma. Those first weeks they'd brought her home she had cowered and hidden, whimpering at the sight of broomsticks. But lately that frozen tentativeness had started to soften. She is playing now, ease creeping back in. We can see it, how something has loosened in her body and, in her new safety, she has bigger things to do than follow orders. Or maybe what she is finally following is herself.

Healing, as we know too well, isn't a linear or even obvious enterprise; we can find evidence of health in a million different subtle signs. But sometimes, returning to our bodies can look like this: more freedom, sovereignty, less obedience to outside rules. Fewer fucks to give, we might say.

So much in the world right now is on fire: the toxicity of systems that incarcerate, control, demolish, diminish. We could get lost in the sorrow. Sometimes, we do.

But then a disobedient dog shows us how to live connected to our inner compass rather than those external obligations. Shows what can be repaired in the face of real safety and abiding love. Sits with her beaming body in a pool of cool water regardless of what the world asks her to do. She has oriented to her own pleasure and, in her defiance, returns to herself.

Engage the Body

My husband, Jon, calls dogs "saltshakers of joy." Wherever they go, they turn up the flavor of pure, bodied contentment. Whether you are a dog person, a cat person, or not inclined to animals at all, see if you might pepper (or salt!) your day with small acts of joy. These might include defiant lingering, like our friend Smokey, or pauses to orient to something that pleases or delights you.

Write

Following my inner compass . . .

Deepen

In part V, we'll keep following this inner compass, letting it guide us toward new discoveries and the movements, places, and practices that feel better.

PART V

Discovery

Movement. Wider. Softer. Finding third ways.

When we practice the fine art of centering what is well without bypassing what truly isn't, we move toward a more spacious way of being with ourselves. What would feel better from here? What else might be possible? In part V, we explore how to reinvite pleasure into the body and how we can use embodied writing as everyday support, building a creative practice that includes joy.

NOT FIXED

One rainy day in my office, a client told me that they felt better. Much better. They could recover from setbacks more quickly and felt a vitality that had been missing. They'd even caught themselves laughing.

"So, am I fixed now?" they asked plaintively. "And if I am, is it the craniosacral work that's made the difference? Or the embodied writing? Or the dietary changes? Or just random?"

"Hm," I said. "What a good question."

It *was* a good question. When we're sick or depressed or feeling broken in some way, we often want to be *fixed*. Of course we do. It'd be so helpful to know what might lead us, step by step, out of the discomfort. A set of rules we can replicate if (when) things go wrong again.

But English is beautiful sometimes.

Because we can fix as in *repair or mend*. Our water line, the broken coffee mug, the ear of our child's teddy bear.

But fixed is also *fastened in place*. As in stuck. Unmoving.

In this second sense, fixed is actually a good description of what happens when we *aren't* well. Whether we're talking about a group of muscles or a sense of despair, in real ways recovering our health means our work is to become *un*fixed.

We are dynamic, which means that every part of us wants to move. Our limbs, breath, cells, blood, lymph. Bodyworkers know to put their hands in fixed places to support loosening. Once we find evidence of movement, we know we're heading toward vitality. In creative practice, we're not looking for a set of rules so much as the pulse of organic movement that guides us in. Are we surprised? Curious? Compelled? These are green lights whispering *keep going, keep going.*

If our bodies are designed to move, our metaphors for health need upgrading. Perhaps we might see ourselves not as a broken series of symptoms and circumstances but simply as stuck, *fixed,* in certain places. Then we could train our attention on the unfixed nascent movements that signal new possibilities. This approach might take us a little further afield, to include in our conception of health all the ways we feel in flow. What we eat, how we sleep, who we share ourselves with, what we let go, whether we are maintaining a writing practice.

During times I've needed support, the practitioners I've liked best—regardless of what they practiced—never bought into the story that I needed fixing; they let me hold my own power close and trusted something deep and potent within me. In their presence, I felt more like a whole person than a series of broken parts. For me, if *fixed* is a black-and-white graph dividing the okay from the not okay, *unfixed* is a peacock's tail: iridescent, multicolored, changed by the angle of the light. So is my dear client "fixed" now? I'm not sure. I can say that the life they're describing sounds more vital, buoyant, and joyful. Triumphantly *un*fixed.

Over these next chapters, we're bringing this more fluid and dynamic notion of health into our practice. We'll continue to hone the fine art of centering on what is well without bypassing or ignoring what isn't, and we'll explore more spacious ways to companion ourselves that reinvite pleasure and possibility into our bodies.

Practice

UNFIXED

In biodynamic craniosacral therapy, we hold an expansive idea of the breath. There is, of course, the breath of the lungs. But then there are other kinds of breath in which all of the structures of the body fluctuate in a kind of tidal rhythm. It can be fruitful (and fun) to exaggerate these subtle oscillations because they show us how our whole structure cycles through these series of dynamic movements.

Engage the Body

If standing is available to your body, gently come to stand with your arms at your sides, your feet hip distance apart, and your knees soft and easy. Feel free to modify these movements from lying down or sitting.

First, breathe. We'll add to these movements over a series of breath cycles.

- On an inhale, bend your knees, straighten as you exhale. Repeat a few times.
- Then on your next inhale add tilting your head back; as you exhale, drop your chin forward to your chest. Repeat a few times.
- On your next inhale, bend your knees, tilt your head back, and add opening your arms wide, exhaling to drop your head, straighten your legs, and close your arms down by your sides.

Repeat the full sequence a few times:

- Inhale: knees bend, head back, arms open, mouth opens.
- Exhale: legs straighten, chin forward, arms close, mouth closes.

In the stillness afterward, linger in the sensation of tidal rhythm moving every part of your own structure. Notice the aliveness of form.

Write

English has a wonderful array of words that evoke new movement. Set your timer for two minutes and try using any (or all!) of these words as a prompt:

- Crack open
- Root
- Emerge
- Unfurl
- Bloom

Afterward, notice which prompts were your favorites and least favorites. Does this give you any new information about your own preferences for growth and movement? What new discoveries have you made around how your body meets transitions?

Deepen

What moves you? What does movement mean to you? What is moving in your life?

Practice

MARMALADE

The moment after the hospital that pleasure reentered my body, it was on my tongue. In early 2020 I did not know what might be possible again, with my body a rack, with skin both taut and limp, with my limbs unreliable.

Until marmalade.

My love for the orange jam arrived like this: across the Atlantic, with my mother, oranges from Spain or Mexico or Florida, bright and sweet. The roots drawn from the Swedish ability to stop in a moment, simply tasting.

Swedes learning English will often sit up midmeal to declare, "Oh! This was good." "Oj! Det var gott." My mother, who's lived in the US for nearly fifty years, still says it.

"No!" We'd cry, the American-born, "It *is* good. You haven't finished!" But we misunderstood this savoring nostalgia that creates edges around pleasure—remember, even now, when it was so good.

At my grandparents' summerhouse, the adults would stop every few hours, for an unhurried fika, a snack and beverage break. The pleasure they took in coffee accompanied by bread with marmalade or perhaps black currant jam, gooseberries, blueberries, the pucker and tang, the cream of butter and cheese.

My body had forgotten it all, displaced itself. Memory eroded, I could not remember when it was ever good.

In the hospital they had a menu, but when I called down to ask for greens or broccoli, they checked my room number. "504? Oh no, low-fiber diet. Would you like white bread? Creamed spinach?" I hadn't touched these foods in years.

I had the hardboiled egg again and could manage a bite, maybe two. My mouth too full of sores, my belly shrunken.

I had forgotten a body could be a channel for something besides pain. I had forgotten that I might walk or bend or ride in a car without wincing, had forgotten this might be possible.

There was a point in my illness where will was gone. There wasn't enough of me to miss what was or hope for something different. Glass-eyed and wan, I sank to the lowest point, like water. Hunger did not exist. In thirst, it was too much to lift a glass. When Nora wanted to show me a picture, turning my head was too much. "Hold it here," I'd say, "in front of my eyes."

I had forgotten hope, despair, movement, air, language, effort, the absence of effort. I had forgotten sex and food and light, had forgotten the play of sun on water refracting light.

Until friends brought food for us and this small golden jar. Finally, the marmalade arrived, over generations, calling me back. Reigniting, reminding.

Until one morning, this burst of tang and orange, of cream and coffee, of feta, properly, in brine. And salt—from the cheese, from my tears. The memory and reclamation of food in pleasure, food as pleasure. "Oh!" I said, midbite, "this was so good."

Engage the Body

Food can be a rich and luscious site that calls in the senses, unspools memory, and invites us to sit down with what tasted so good. Not only flavor but setting and timing will influence what we taste and remember. What strikes us might be a banquet of crayfish and melted butter or cold dill rice eaten off a paper plate beside a river. As we explore a memory of food, see if you can bring to mind a meal or snack that echoes with sumptuousness in your body.

Write

A food memory that delights you . . .

SPELLCASTING IN THE SILENCE

In the big room at the end of the hall, I was casting spells. Technically, we first graders were sitting in Quaker Meeting for Worship, the "silent meeting" that our class endured every Wednesday, when all of us gathered together to sit quietly in what was intended to be a period of reverent communion with spirit. But I, with my bowl cut and button-up shirt, was pantomiming a great performance to my friend Hannah across the room, in which I was a witch and the circle was a cauldron. I flung my arms wide to reach for frogs' legs and eye of newt, then stirred the potion in dramatic circles with a great, invisible spoon.

I felt a firm hand on my leg. My teacher, Bisse, Swedish like my mother, only a sturdier version, with clacking bracelets and short hair, whispered seriously: "BROWN BENCH, JOHANNA."

I headed over to the bench of exile in the corner, away from the staring six- and seven-year-olds still on the rug. Never mind, I would continue to concoct my magic potions from over there.

As a child in the Quaker school where my mother was also a teacher, meeting for worship was a weekly ritual I detested. The enforced silence took my boredom to new and deeper levels of intolerability for which I devised ever more creative ways to disrupt the interminable quiet.

Outside of silent meetings, I loved school. The building, a bizarre relic of '60s modernist architecture, sat on the footprint of an old pottery factory, leaving us great clay pits to muck about in whenever it rained. We wrote and performed operas, painted giant murals across the playground, and delved deep in music class, performing gospel, discordant Bulgarian songs, and Frank Zappa. Rarely did we notice the explicitly Quaker parts of our education, but there were a few notable exceptions. Quakers make decisions by consensus rather than voting, which meant that we spent all of third grade debating the names of our class hamsters. It's possible my memory has embellished this story, but when—after months—we all finally agreed to the names Kit Kat and Hershey, the rodents promptly died, offering us important lessons in civics, compromise, and bereavement. As we got older, our schooling included multiday workshops on prejudice and racism, curricula that examined histories of oppression, architectures of privilege, and our responsibilities in speaking truth to power. In the heady days of 1980s Cambridge, Massachusetts, the work wasn't called social justice, but it shared the same DNA.

It was years before I realized that silent meeting wasn't separate from our work in the world, but fundamental to it. These containers of shared quiet fueled a clarity of purpose and connection. "A Quaker meeting," says educator and writer Parker Palmer, "is meant to be a live encounter from which arises real work and real life."[16] The silence in meeting wasn't a passive final destination but a precursor to right action.

Sitting in stillness to inform the next movement isn't unique to Quakerism. Other traditions call us to prayer, or meditation, or chanting, or any number of practices that listen in a wider way. When I began biodynamic craniosacral work, I recognized the cultivation of this engaged, present space from which new possibilities might arise, paths my grasping mind could never imagine.

Part of what I came to love about this stillness and space was that it was available regardless of our condition. When we're sick or stuck, overwhelmed or underresourced, it calls us inward. From here, we might find solace in a Quaker phrase that's recruited when the path forward is opaque: *Way will open.* The saying invites sitting in the discomfort of not knowing to listen for a choice or pathway that hasn't yet revealed itself. *Way will open* isn't passive waiting so much as active, curious listening.

Not that sitting in uncertainty is a picnic. And there are times when way, stubbornly, *doesn't* open. But that too can be instructive. Palmer writes of an elder who said, "In sixty-plus years of living, way has never opened in front of me . . . But a lot of way has closed behind me, and that's had the same guiding effect."[17]

Here in our embodied writing practice, we're getting closer to the stillness that precedes action, feeling into the delicate balance between acceptance and change, and listening through our bodies to recognize the somatic pulse of *way opening* into new ways forward. And yes, friends, we are casting spells. Not with eye of newt but with witness, with creating, with imagination, with care.

Practice

ADORNING THE EMPTINESS

Sometimes the move from one state to another can be the difference of just a few degrees. From the outside no one else would likely recognize the shift, but when something imbues the space we're in with compassion, or curiosity, or beauty it can transform empty loneliness into tranquil solitude.

In workshops I like to call in writer Toko-pa Turner's words on cultivating magic inside the emptiness. She writes,

> This is the true meaning of prayer. To clear an emptiness in our lives where the holy can enter. To prepare a place in our home, in our lives, in our hearts, where magic can feel welcome. And while nothing happens for an uncomfortable amount of time, we can adorn that emptiness with the humble images of our own longing.[18]

In this practice, we're taking inspiration from Turner to let our longing bloom inside empty spaces.

Engage the Body

See if you might create a space of quiet inside yourself by letting your shoulders drop, loosening your belly, and taking a few slow breaths. In the stillness that follows, consider how you might fill this space with beauty, with longing, with metaphor or image.

Write

Adorn the emptiness . . .

FIRST PERSON

In the Emptiness

Erika Arthur describes herself as "in training to be a human being, apprenticed primarily, but not exclusively, to teachers who are more than human." In our embodied writing workshop, she explored the prompt adorn the emptiness . . .

EMPTINESS

I hang your old shirt on the nail
                    in the emptiness,
not for practicality or decoration,
but as an invitation—
come visit sometimes,
come as your softest self,
the one I used to sleep in
when I was small.
I light a candle
                    in the emptiness,
not for light to read by
or small warmth,
but for magic—
when you're here
we'll dance on the walls
to the beat of one small drum.
I leave my shoes at the door
                    of the emptiness,
not to keep it clean
of sand and salt,
or out of piety
or duty,

but so I can feel
the texture
                    of the emptiness.

This poem was written in an embodied writing workshop in the months after my father took his own life at the age of sixty-eight. Some part of me must have known this grief was not going to be an above-the-shoulders process and I was going to need some accompaniment, because I signed up for the workshop even though I had no idea what it would be like, especially online in the early-pandemic days.

In retrospect I can see that in a way, my father's death freed me from the kind of thinking I am deeply habituated to and released me into the viscerality of deep loss. Embodied writing practice helped me realize this. Receiving generous guidance to tap into the body as part of the writing process helped me integrate fragments of image, memory, and sensation that were emerging unbidden during this period. It gave me some small ways to be my own witness through the uncharted territory of the loss of a parent to suicide.

Entering my writing through the door of the body revealed some surprising new metaphors. Sometimes the body can produce its own medicine when I can, with care, invite language to emerge from embodied experience. In turn, it can reveal something that feels true, even if unexpected or unfamiliar. And that truth can be a tender companion, even if only momentarily.

Practice

PERSPECTIVE SHIFT

Once, looking out from the attic window at the trees outside, I swore I saw, in the flecks of sun catching the light, filaments of the largest spiderweb on earth.

You've maybe had those moments too. You're walking through the woods or a field, and you see light moving along strands in midair, suddenly making visible the lines of a web.

But . . . from up here? How was it possibly discernible from this distance? Was this the strangest, strongest, longest spiderweb of all time?

Until, shifting my focus to the pond beyond the trees, I realized the fluttering light was dozens of birds, the sun catching their bodies like bits of gold. Not the web of a spider but a different kind of web entirely, alive in movement. *Ohhhhh.* I gasped in surprise.

I needed the gift of this image.

The day before, I had sat with a friend who was navigating late-stage cancer. I marveled at the stream of family and friends that came through: the bakery owner next door, a high school friend, his dad downstairs. Sometimes the phrase *we are here for you* isn't an abstraction but an urgent truth wrapped in grief and love. Each of us was trying to find ways to turn our despair into labor or service while we could.

When I can't find words or my small human mind starts grasping, I try to look for clues in the world around me. Sometimes, if I'm lucky, I stumble on treasure.

Because those golden birds *were* a web but an unexpected one. To see it required shifting my perspective to recognize a different kind of connection, one threaded not through fixed lines but the bodies themselves, engaged in acts of care and love, the strands only visible when the light was just right.

Engage the Body

Perspective shifts can turn the kaleidoscope on our view of the world, bringing new color and shape to the frame. Here, we play with subtle shifts of the eyes to notice different kinds of focus.

Begin by closing your eyes and letting them rest. Next, open your eyes and choose an object in the room to focus on (plant, sock, mug—anything will do). Focus all your attention here for a few breaths, then, softening your focus, widen out your attention to include the periphery. Play with moving back and forth from focusing to widening, noticing how the rest of your body feels as you subtly shift your gaze through these different kinds of noticing.

Write

How I see it . . .

RÉVÉRENCE

One Saturday morning I found myself with twelve other women, stretching on yoga mats in front of the campus vending machines. Together, we were a sea of spandex and tight cotton. We breathed into our bellies, stretching and moving our spines in all directions.

"So," Claudette turned to me brightly, "are we ready to write?" Claudette Ndayininahaze is one of the directors of In Her Presence, a group she co-founded with Abusana "Micky" Bondo to help immigrant women grow their collective empowerment. Their organization offers English classes, employment, childcare, and an entire array of options to meet an array of needs. On any given Saturday, you might find refugee and immigrant women in rich conversation on poetry, job applications, health and healthcare, and history. Today, embodied writing. I looked out at the group.

"Okay!" I said. "We're going to play with writing and moving today, but this isn't school. You don't have to worry about grammar or spelling. We'll give ourselves permission to play, to see where we go." Someone said the word *permission* in Arabic. We talked about listening with reverence. A pause to check on French translation. "Oui," said someone in blue, "just the same, révérence."

After introductions and stretching, we had time for one writing prompt: *I remember.* I reminded the group to be gentle and slow with themselves in the exercise. The room went quiet with the scribbling of pencils, all of us bent over our notebooks, remembering. When it was time to share, Olivia, a grandmother from Iraq in a yellow scarf, declared with a laugh, "Remember! What is this 'remember'? We come here to FORGET." Celine, from Burundi, wrote about the contents of her fridge while Aya shared the talk she had with her mother that morning, still in Damascus. We listened and laughed, nodded and wept, each of us recognizing parts of ourselves in each other's stories.

The spark of these moments in workshops kindled something. It didn't seem to matter who we were or where we came from or what we believed. Our bodies contained our stories, we were willing to share them, and breathing permission suffused the writing and listening. Together we felt the mercy and exultation of extending ourselves in vulnerability and being met with kind witness.

The more I shared embodied writing, the more it worked its magic back on me. Something was happening in those rooms. At barns in Freeport and flamenco studios in Portland, at art programs for adults with disabilities, yurts in Cumberland, and cancer centers in Scarborough. People walked out trusting something new within them, among them.

I couldn't quite name what was opening up in these spaces. There was the writing and the moving, there was tenderness and laughter and sharing. But what was this nascent feeling that kept showing up? Perhaps the repair of a split I'd carried between what I felt and what I shared. In these spaces, we could let loose, speak true, feel what we felt. Whatever I offered through these workshops was returning something doubly, a fullness I didn't have courage for at the beginning of illness, an experience of letting it all belong.

Practice

LOVE IS SPACE

Becoming a biodynamic craniosacral therapist changed my practice and my life. *Presence without scrutiny* became a guiding principle of my work, and I'd watch as clients settled from a feeling of buzzing activation into a more peaceful state. And not just more peaceful—the work was never to banish hurt or insist on calm—but connected to a deeper well of capacity, one that let them meet the moment with a greater sense of resource and trust. After years of trying to "help" clients feel better, it was almost frustrating to see how much more effective it was to drop the notion of helping altogether and simply listen with a spacious and abiding presence. Of course I wanted clients to feel better, but when I committed to companioning them inside their discomfort rather than needing them to overcome it, the results were body-centered and longer lasting.

Later, I learned a new name for this engaged, present, permissive space: love. The Rev. angel Kyodo williams describes this elegantly in an interview from *On Being*:

> The way that I think of love most often these days is that love is space . . . to come from a place of love is to be in acceptance of what is, even in the face of moving it towards something that is more whole, more just, more spacious for all of us.[19]

Perhaps that was why practicing felt so good; it was a kind of heart-centered generosity that made room for whatever arose. Love as a way of listening alongside our many other essential needs: medical care and medicine, access to nature, nutrition, places to rest, safety.

I wanted to better understand *love is space*, so I turned to my dear friend, psychiatrist and psychoanalyst Dr. Megan Poe. Megan taught New York University's popular love class and is an artist, musician, and all-round galactic human. "Love is the natural order of things," Megan explained. The medium and the bass note of the universe. It's also radically connective and "teaches us to be in relationship to people, nature, the more-than-human world, art, objects, songs." She suggested that we might simply follow the advice of the poet Rumi and look for the barriers we've created against love.

On the wrong frequency, "holding space" might feel like an empty phrase. But if it's space imbued and engaged with love, space that doesn't look away from what hurts, it's actually what Megan calls *a strategy and a solvent.* "Love appears and what was impossible is now possible." Unlike the mental body, whose solutions involve getting away from whatever *this* is, love does not run from the reality we're living inside of. It has the capacity to both accept what's here and tug on the thread of future possibilities that are, as Rev. angel says, "more whole, more just, more spacious for all of us." This is where our work in reverent listening, permission, and widening range bears fruit: We're honing a more inclusive way of understanding health, one generous enough to say to whatever mood, illness, rupture, or yearning arrives on the scene, *there's space for you too.*

Engage the Body

Notice what happens in your body when you hear the word *spacious.* Do your shoulders fall, even slightly? Does your chest widen? To deepen into this feeling you might imagine yourself floating on your back or gazing up at a sky full of stars. Once you feel like you've connected with this sense of wide-openness, see if you might offer this kind of allowing, flexible presence to yourself. Take a moment to notice what arises, feeling your breath, shoulders, discomforts, cravings—allowing spaciousness to imbue all of it.

Write

With enough space . . .

Deepen

Get curious about what love means to you. For inspiration, you might find the recording of Wendell Berry reading his poem, "The Peace of Wild Things." Then write into *love is* . . . This might be a list or a piece of paper you keep in your pocket as you move through your day, finding examples of love. An excellent beat that you hear from a passing car? The concentration of a toddler working his way through an ice cream? A generous and unremarkable act, like a door held open or a blanket folded? All might be examples of love.

Practice

WHAT WOULD FEEL BETTER?

Sometimes we facilitators need someone else to hold our hand through a process. On a spring evening marked by a classic Maine mix of pink blossoms and frigid air, I met up with my friend Sage Hayes to discuss this very book. We walked a loop past the bridge park with its giant concrete columns and out beyond the car dealerships.

Sage is a deeply skilled somatics facilitator who practices embodied presence and relational care. They're also someone I love and trust, with a knack for helping folks shift the whole frame. On this night, as I wrung my hands about how to feel my way into this book, this book I'd been writing and rewriting for nearly a decade, they offered a simple, potent practice.

Sage stopped on the sidewalk. "Here," they said, "put out your hands. What does this book feel like?" I reached my hands into the air, imagining I was holding this book. It was blue, light filled, like a copse of trees or a walk through a garden at twilight. The book felt easy, a gentle way of arriving.

"Okay," they said. "Now lean into this process of creating the book, lean into the discomfort and feel that."

There on the sidewalk, I leaned into the distinct feeling that I had no idea what I was doing: sparks in my chest, dizziness. It *wasn't* comfortable, but I stayed with it, feeling both the overwhelm and the excitement.

"Now, see if you can make some move towards what would feel better. Listen in your body for how you might move from here. Up? To the side? Backwards?"

Holding my imaginary book it felt so clear: inward, downward. I brought my hands in toward my body, lowered them slightly. Everything felt a little quieter now, more settled.

"Good," Sage said. "Now notice from here what shape or form surrounds you. What else do you see?"

I suddenly noticed golden hexagons in the air around us, as though we were surrounded by a hive of support. Fascinating. We moved on to other topics, but the image and feeling lingered with me.

When I got home, I drew the hexagonal cell of a hive encircled by the words "shape of a session / shape of a class" and recognized that the organic structure of the book *already* existed. I had been living this process since the beginning: We arrive and begin with acknowledgments, settle and meet, offer permission, reverence, witness. We take inventory, check in, name and grieve and allow. Doing so makes us wider and softer, until we begin to discover that we can move through this together, forming a coherent inclusive collective of individual stories, an emergence. Rinse and repeat; we begin again. The six-part structure of this book comes from that night on the sidewalk, guiding me to a deeper frame that I could somatically feel.

Sage facilitated a conversation between the present and future, a back and forth guided by imagination and subtle body shifts that helped me reorient to choice and pleasure. It was a profound process that hinged on the simple question: What would feel better from here?

Engage the Body

Bring to mind a place in your life that feels stuck or overwhelmed. This might be a project or a situation or a relationship—any area that doesn't have the signature of ease. Begin by noticing how this feels in your body, staying with however the discomfort presents itself. Then get curious about *what would feel better from here.* Not as an idea or a solution but as a literal movement you might make in space. Try letting that feeling express itself in a body shift in some direction. Up? To the right? Deep underground? Once you've located a small shift that feels better, widen out the field to notice if any other images or shapes are present here.

Write

Narrate your experience of this exercise. What feels better from here? What new shapes or images present themselves? What does this process show you?

THE FULLNESS OF YOUR OWN ECOSYSTEM

Perhaps you know the feeling: On the outside, things look fine ("fine"—beware this menacing word that often glosses over what definitely isn't). You're functioning and doing what needs to be done. The dishes are cleanish, and the kids are getting fed, and no one at work is complaining.

But.

When you slow down enough to feel how you actually are, a very different sort of picture: desolate, alone, crisped, dizzy. You're spinning somewhere off in the dark.

An exhale. A pause.

You might, if you tilt your head and squint, recognize that you aren't describing a living body so much as a moon. This place, this version of you, is devoid of gravity, caught in the orbit of the planets that surround you. Whatever matters is somewhere else. Life itself is elsewhere. Subtly and without meaning to, you have become someone who moves around what others need, existing in response to life, someplace far away.

But friends, let us call this the lie that it is. You are not a moon to everyone else's needs but a wildly beautiful, complex planet. Your own whole, gorgeous ecosystem. Teeming with life. Oxygenated. Perhaps you might remember the fullness of your own ecosystem and allow this recognition to return you to yourself. Over the years, I've watched this small acknowledgment reset a sense of holding in countless clients.

My wise Nora, when I shared this metaphor with her, pointed out that planets *also* exist in orbits, but larger ones, around the sun. She's right, of course. And with her help we might take this further: We *are* moving together, part of a vast galactic whole. But we can cultivate intimacy and interdependence without draining ourselves of resources. The universe has plenty of space for our vast complexity, our seasons and terrains, our flora and fauna.

I've found that this reorientation isn't necessarily visible to the outside. We may appear the same, working as much and washing the same dishes, but inside we're holding the truth that our actual life is here, on our own planet. This is an entire world to inhabit, one full of mystery, with its own wise pacing. Its own particular rhythms. This is you, beloved.

Practice

FEELING YOUR OWN SPINE

In this practice, we're deepening into the axis at our center; letting our attention come from the potency of this great organizing midline.

Engage the Body

Find a foam body roller or use a rolled-up towel or yoga mat so that you have access to a long, soft cylinder.

- Sitting up with your sacrum anchored to the base of the cylinder, begin by mobilizing the spine—flexing and extending, rocking, swaying.
- With much gentleness, come to rest in a supine (face-up) position, so that the length of your spine is supported along the length of this soft cylinder, keeping knees bent, and arms extended at your sides or resting on your torso.
- What do you notice as you seat your attention in your midline?
- Stay as long as it feels good and exit by gently rolling to one side.

Write

My spine . . .

Deepen

Imagine this spine is the central axis of your own planet, an entire world to inhabit, one full of mystery and its own particular rhythms. What might it look like to inhabit your own ecosystem? To practice living less like a moon orbiting others and more like a planet in your own right?

Practice
SIGNS OF LIFE

2008. I had been out of the hospital for a few months and was slowly recovering. One early morning, when the moon was still up, I walked down to the pond through the dark trees, the air chilled and milky. Quiet. Five deer scared through the tall grass, their white tails like waving apostrophes. There was the crackle of my footsteps on dry leaves through the field, the split of sticks as I entered the forest, bramble catching on my pant legs. Still hushed.

But as I came up over the rise there was a call, four notes, and then another, a trilling robin, and soon the air was only song. Red-winged blackbird, plaintive chickadee. Mourning dove, starling. The harsh squawk of blue jays and crows. Everywhere, from above and beside and beneath. A bath of sound. Then, a splash. From my perch on the rock I saw a muskrat moving quickly away from the reeds, a large fanning v trailing behind, the ripples turning silver as they caught the light of dawn, like mercury set free.

The world, I thought, is animate. *Not in spite of these bodies but because of them.* I had been trying for so long to avoid the truth of this, pretending to be constituted by effort and determination alone. Ashamed of my failing body, I'd treated it as a side project, an inconvenient asterisk beside the things that mattered: my job, my responsibilities. The hubris of all this suddenly seemed like a bad joke, like being sucker punched by my own stubborn delusion.

What if, arrived the question, I let in the truth of my body's condition? Could there be a way of resting in what was actually here? And what if I were still enough, even broken? Touching this possibility felt thrilling, like discovering a new language. In relinquishing the veneer of being okay, I began to discover, beneath all that muck, the radiance of my actual health.

Engage the Body

From the bottom of the ravine, life can feel very spare and still. I've found enormous solace in parking lot weeds pushing asphalt aside to demand their time in the sun. Particles of dust that play in the light, irrespective of gravity. Lichen on rocks that seem too barren to support life, and yet.

Today, we're looking for evidence of life, and we're casting a wide net. Not a glib exercise in gratitude, but a scientific collection of data: Where is the world animate? Where am *I* animate? Notice from right here, or take yourself on a walk and bring your notebook along.

Write

Evidence of life . . .

Use your notebook to create a list or a brief catalog.

Deepen

Choose one sign of life from your list, and see if you can practice feeling that pulse or movement or expression in your own body. Perhaps you might sketch this movement or create a poem inspired by what you saw.

Practice

HOW TO LOVE YOUR BODY

When friend, writer, and mentor Susan Conley offered our writing group the prompt *how to love your body*, I balked. *Did she say love your body?* What fantasy world would I have to recruit to even entertain this question?

Many of us don't have much practice loving our bodies. Particularly if you are assigned female at birth (AFAB), you've probably been taught by society at large to regard your body from the outside, picking and critiquing. If you are bedbound or diseased and it feels like your body is what's keeping you from life, summoning love might feel especially challenging.

For me, compiling a set of instructions on how to love your body felt like a real stretch.

But then, sinking in, something happened.

"How to" prompts are sneakily generative. They recruit a part of us that instructs, pulling us out of the muck and turning us toward a larger circle. Cooking dinner every night can be a drag, but when my daughter enters the kitchen and wants to make soup? Suddenly, I've taken interest in every part. *Begin with the big knife; no, use this one. Grab the carrots, onions, celery—a fine dice, like this. Now heat the pot slowly; let the flavors build.* And I'm off. Reignited.

When Susan offered us *how to love your body*, this guiding teacher part of me sparked to attention. I actually could recover memories of loving this body, could recognize moments of delight and freedom. As I let myself deepen into the exploration, my "body" grew to include different terrains. Earth body. Bodies of water. My mental body playing with words and phrases. Oh! I could tell you how to love so many of these bodies. What came out was a tumble, a very specific set of memories and instructions:

> *Leave the country; don't look back. Surround yourself with queer uncles who both adore you and cannot be bothered with you. Stain your hands with*

> *blueberries. Sing, full-throated at the table, words you don't yet understand. Eat. Eat cakes, eat sour milk, cracker bread by the packageful. Undress in the yellow room upstairs, heading out to the sauna where your uncle enthusiastically throws water on the walls and stove, making steam that burns, purges, stifles and finally, the discomfort building to a crescendo, sends you out, slamming the door behind you, into the lake, steam rising from your body, the sky light at 10:30 p.m., a peace in you that is singular and total, that could not happen without this body, that could not happen anywhere but here.*

Susan's prompt created an exquisite loop, from body to page and back again. In part III we explored writer Melissa Febos's words on rolling back the tape to a time when she felt the "perfect freedom of caring about only what my body could do and never how it was seen." The passage ends with another gem: "Loving myself has never been something I was able to do simply by deciding to. It is something I learned to do through intensive self-reflection. Through writing and making art. Through a close study of what brings me joy and gives my life meaning."[20] Recalling moments when I loved this body lit this vital connection between writing, reflecting, living, and embodiment that is at the heart of our practice here.

Engage the Body

Invite yourself to get wide, easy, and soft. Shift into a lens that looks lovingly, without correction of any kind. Get free ranging, fantastical, understanding *body* in any way that is currently resonant for you.

Write

How to love your body . . .

Practice

LIMINAL

At some point in my process of learning to live with chronic disease, I arrived at the mysterious gap between my old ways of operating and new ways of being that were still forming. Perhaps you've also visited this strange zone that is the hallmark of transformation. Liminality: the phase in the middle, when we're no longer recognizable as who we were, and we're not fully developed into what we're becoming.

Which perhaps sounds poetic, but in real life can feel excruciatingly disorienting. Particularly since regular life doesn't generally offer acknowledgment or rituals that might support us in moving from one stage to another, liminality can feel muddy and deeply questioning. Something inside is shifting, but—now what? Faced with uncertainty in this bizarre middle place, we might find ourselves casting about frantically, asking questions like *What am I supposed to do with my life now?* Or *maybe I should move / change jobs / go back to school / end this relationship.* Mostly, the essence of all this *what do I do?* boils down to *who am I now?*

But, friends, not knowing means *we haven't been here before.* Which tells us we're growing. And while there can be a kind of frustrated indignity—wasn't all this waking up supposed to make me feel better?—if we have the temerity to hang out here without rushing an answer, our bodies will show us some deep and simple truths. Guidance we won't recognize if we're in the urgency of figuring it out.

I wish my experience here came from the cool distance of research instead of the messy trenches. Waking up to my body doesn't always feel better, but it does allow me to feel. And that is itself a kind of roadmap, showing what tugs at curiosity and often—after a choice of some kind—what truly doesn't. In my messy twenties, my wise friend Bill told me I was going through a necessary precursor to adulthood: "learning to flail."

Here in our unfolding practice, we have a lot of tools for meeting this pause. Writing. Moving. Following the inner compass toward what is beautiful or interesting. Staying as resourced as we can. Feeling into our deeper rhythms, or bodied breath. Not rushing to fix or even comprehend this bizarre middle zone. Perhaps even a bit of faith that way will open. To be in the pause asks for gentleness and invites mystery. We can remind each other to include *permission and reverence.* To keep showing up.

Engage the Body

Spend a few minutes in quiet, slow breath. See if you can include a lengthening pause between each in-breath and out-breath. Let your shoulders drop, your belly soften, and notice how this in-between space feels.

Write

In the pause . . . What do you notice in this liminal between place? This still point of potency? See where the writing takes you.

Practice

IN PRAISE OF THE UNNECESSARY

One early summer, a bird woke me up every morning at a little past four. The singing was relentlessly cheerful. Also loud.

Go back to bed, I murmured. Is this really necessary?

Ah, "necessary." Behind this innocent-seeming word is a whole framework we might not detect, so early in the morning, one that insists on being reasonable, that decides what matters, which is not this. What is necessary can lead to a kind of brutalist architecture of life: work, eat, sleep, repeat.

I have absolutely squandered opportunities for joy in the name of the necessary.

In my twenties, I showed up to a Halloween party in the Berkshires wearing jeans and an old sweater. My friend Matthew, assessing my outfit, asked kindly, "Jonesy, where is your costume?" "Oh," I explained. "I don't do dress-up. I've outgrown that nonsense." And then he took my hands, looked at me seriously, and said, "We are going to change all that right now. We're going to create a ridiculous costume for you, and you will never look back." We pulled something together, and I danced through that night in a resplendent whirl of pink and glitter and face paint.

Years on, my closet now includes sequins and wigs and wings for all manner of occasion. Are they necessary? Not a single bit. Have they provided fuel for spontaneous parades and dance parties? Certainly. All this may sound careless, silly, unserious. And friends, it is. Getting out from under necessary opens a rich field of possibilities that contains the germ of your true responsibility: the care and keeping of your one wild and precious life. Claiming playfulness without apology, without earning it through work or obligation, lands us in the softer place where things grow.

I have spent months on the floor of the bathroom, too sick to move, drained of all will. If someone had pranced in suggesting playfulness, I would have had some choice words. Also gestures. When you are trying to survive, life shrinks to what is necessary. But if you start to feel your margins grow, whimsy is the tell of true health. A secret signal that life is animate, surprising, and sometimes even fun.

Engage the Body

What is one easy, pleasurable, and absolutely unnecessary action you might offer yourself today? Perhaps it's a different route home. A lit candle. A body wrapped in something warm. Copying a poem you love in your notebook. These actions require no spending of money at all; we're simply seeding joy.

Write

Sometimes it is necessary . . .

LAGOM

The lists can seem so innocent. "Once I have time," they begin, and after that, a litany: I'll exercise more, reach out to that friend I've been meaning to contact, organize the bathroom, research the medication, do that thing and make that thing and clean that thing . . .

Unremarkable, right? Until you notice how tightly you've been holding yourself, how packed in it all feels. All those lists can create a kind of quiet patina of self-scolding over a subtext that is clear and sharp: *Be better. Get better. Do better*. Call it late-stage capitalism, call it a legacy of colonialism and exploitation, but this drone of never-ending self-improvement insidiously ties our value to what we can show for it. Which can wreak havoc on your sense of self-worth and belonging.

But it doesn't have to be this way. And in some places, it isn't.

At my family's house in Sweden, every dinner was followed by dessert. And nearly every dessert was whittled down, bit by bit, cut in half infinitely like a Zeno's paradox of cake, until only a small nub remained. The nub went in the fridge, where it generally remained until it was time for the compost.

No one would take that last bite.

Maybe this sounds wasteful, self-denying, and silly. Why not grab the laurels of dessert for yourself? But it was part of an ethos that knows we're all sharing the same cake. No one is more entitled or special than anyone else. It's a belief encapsulated by the Swedish idea of lagom.

Lagom is difficult to translate into English, because we immediately bump into a whole set of values: In the US, when we say something is *enough* or *average* or *appropriate,* it connotes a bummer of a situation. In a country built on a legacy of taking, anything less than all isn't good enough. But lagom follows a different frame in which everyone is equally deserving, regardless of what they've accomplished or made. The size of our portion needs to be in proportion to a whole. The lagom-sized piece isn't the biggest, it's whatever size ensures everyone can eat.* It feels so much less precarious, to trust you'll receive an equal portion of dessert, regardless of how bedbound, unproductive, or exceptional you are.

Perhaps the real injury underneath those to-do lists is how much their determined betterment separates us from the larger whole. Right at the moment when connection might actually help us feel better, our determination to *be better* creates small silos of exceptionality, cutting us off from the very thing we need.

What might happen if we allowed ourselves to be honest about what dwells inside, offering permission instead of improvement? Getting low and close with these tender places nests us in a kinder and more inclusive lagom, one that doesn't require a better version of us but simply knows we belong.

---

* There's nuance to lagom, which applies not just to dessert but also to temperatures, feelings, things, situations, and sometimes temperaments. And while I've seen lagom trend as a fix for capitalistic greed, I've also experienced it as a repressive concept around behavior. I embrace my freak, as do my friends and family; we will not be tamping down our too muchness to fit in. Let us borrow the parts of lagom that resonate.

Practice

WHAT MATTERS

Sometimes, the best cure for holding too tight is to remember what feels truly important. In this practice, we get real with what matters. We remember our vast planetary-ness and connect with what I think of as the holy trinity:

- We *are* matter.
- We *do* matter.
- We are *held by* the great mater (the great mother).

Each of these affirmations supports the others, creating a kind of webbed support. You are earthy and bodied, literally matter. Your life, however it's expressing itself, is a gift: *you* matter. We are sustained and kept alive by this beneficent earth, our magna mater (our *great mother*).

Engage the Body

Practice holding this trinity of mattering. First feel your bones, skin, hands. Feel your weight and gravity. Then feel for your spine as a potent, vertical axis, down into the earth, and up through your crown into sky. Finally, widen your field to notice the earth mother/mater beneath, around, above, and through you.

Write

What matters . . .

Practice

SISTER VESSELS

Sometimes our grief circles the places we didn't go and the people we did not become. Acknowledging these other lives can help us find new softness for the path we did end up on.

In "The Blue House," poet Tomas Tranströmer writes beautifully about how we can simultaneously feel gratitude for the life we have and yearn for the paths not taken. In this practice, we're following Tranströmer's lead to make space for the ghost ships and sister vessels of lives not led.

Write

The multiverse is a common device in sci-fi movies, a way of showing those parallel and alternate lives we could have lived. Take a few moments imagining these other worlds, perhaps as ghost ships following other routes. *What might your life look like with a different body, choice, universe?*

ORGANIC IGNITION (WHAT READINESS LOOKS LIKE)

Back at Good Medicine Collective, dusk was settling over Casco Bay. Early spring's return meant a later sunset, and we oohed and ahhed at the returning light. Tonight we were exploring a new concept. I looked around the circle to explain.

"We often initiate action from *have to*. Dinner needs making. Laundry must be folded. Work or family or household requires . . . something." Lara nodded her head. Kate sighed in recognition. "Which means that most of us aren't often practicing activity that engages because curiosity or beauty or some nameless feeling compels us to move." I paused to make sure this landed with the group. "Tonight we're exploring movement that isn't coerced but ignites on its own—we can call this *organic ignition*."

In biodynamic craniosacral therapy we're interested in the energy that precedes matter. We listen for conditions that arise *before* movement is even visible. So I wanted to see if our group might explore what combination of factors come together to compel movement. What impulse or feeling might carry us across the threshold from bud to blossom?

"I'm not so sure about readiness," said Eleanor. "It never feels that smooth for me."

"Me neither," said Ayanna. "Spring is sold as this blooming beauty, but that isn't my experience of transition at all."

Outside the window, muddy snowbanks were a good reminder that spring itself—that symbol of awakening—doesn't begin with joyful easy opening but can be a sloppy mess, full of stops and starts. Same goes for the ocean; when the tide goes slack, it's a disorganized state. Some parts ebbing, others flowing. In the marshes, things get turbid and weird. No wonder Five Element acupuncturists describe the emotional energy of spring as anger. That irritated feeling that *this is now too small for me* can propel a seed into a sprout, but getting there isn't necessarily comfortable or smooth.

There are seasonal ignitions and then there's also this: When we're deeply depleted, the notion of moving again can feel not just awkward but beyond even imagining.

In my late twenties I had to take a leave from work because an ongoing flare of my disease had reduced me to a brittle twig. Despite a strict program of bed rest, three weeks later I could still barely move. I felt like a sieve through which vitality passed but did not stay. Truthfully, I didn't even want more energy, *I wanted to want* more energy.

My doctor at the time was a kind woman who drew a line on a scrap of paper, high and straight. "You have been running on adrenaline," she said, gesturing at the paper. "But that was false energy." Here she drew her pen down, creating a precipitous drop-off. "And now you don't have it. Your gauges are broken, and your tanks are empty. It'll take time to rebuild." I hated hearing this.

But then months later, smelling a blooming lilac in the yard, I realized with a start that I had made my way outside *because I wanted to and I could*. There was finally enough capacity and a true desire to go. Movements that arise organically cannot be coerced and aren't necessarily grand gestures. I've never found my way there by figuring it out or overriding my exhaustion. It was more like trusting the breathing dynamic between movement and resting, each essential to the other.

The sun was passing beneath the horizon now, and I dimmed the lights in the big room and invited the group to lie down and get comfortable with blankets and props. Before writing, we would explore listening for the readiness that precedes movement. Maybe you'd like to join us?

Practice

READINESS

Here we're listening for what compels our whole system—heart, body, spirit, mind—to find its rhythm.

Engage the Body

Create a comfortable place to lie down, perhaps dimming the lights or placing a cloth over your eyes. Begin by taking a few deep breaths and allowing yourself a full-body stretch, extending toes and arms in opposite directions. Feel the support of whatever is beneath you and let your limbs and torso sink into rest.

Then imagine you're a seed, tucked in the earth, deep in winter's exhalation. From here, consider what offers you real and resting comfort, what objects or spaces or resources give you a sense of relief and reassurance. After a few breaths, transition to imagining what might compel you to move. What are foods or places, textures or experiences that delight or nourish you, tug you toward them or encourage an extending reach? For a seed this might be sunshine, rain, or an internal *time to go*. A human, meanwhile, might be more compelled by an excellent cup of coffee or an irresistible beat. Could your curiosity, love, or compassion help you discern a spark of ignition?

Feel free to play here in the subtle body, moving between a sense of rooting down into comfort and growing outward in curiosity. What do you notice about what happens *before* you feel ready to move?

Write

Before I begin . . .

PART VI

Connection. Collective. Song.

With a more robust sense of language and practice, we widen out to see the ways in which we are fundamentally supported, alive, and accompanied. Whether in human community or the living world, we begin to attend to the circulation of resource in a larger sense.

Part VI explores putting it all together: How do we live as well as we can with the bodies, histories, and sensitivities we have? How do we locate choice and space amid the demands of life? The care and keeping of an embodied writing practice helps.

CROWN SHYNESS

In November of 2019, after a long period of quiet, my autoimmune disease slowly dismantled all the structures of my life. The craniosacral practice I loved, the people I wanted to see, the public events that lifted my spirits, everything went silent as illness became all encompassing. First housebound and then hospital bound, I spent most of December, January, and February recuperating. I joked with friends that I was earning a black belt in convalescence and a gold medal in lying around.

I never thought this would be useful.

Until, just at the moment I was ready to return to life, the coronavirus arrived. Nora called it "world cancellation." We were all so blindsided by this confusing, upside-down landscape: We needed one another but had to be separate. We had time and space but no assurance of income. We were all so alone, together. However the pandemic imploded in your own life, you likely remember this time well.

But if being housebound taught me anything, it was to look outside, to find solace in nature even if you aren't actually able to go there. Which is why I turned to trees.

As a broad collective, trees are some of our greatest teachers. Rooting deep while reaching upward, trees send messages via underground mycorrhizal networks, constantly transmitting and receiving information through the microcosmos. They are generous with their elders and nurturing of their young sprouts, sharing nutrients as well as information about predators and disease. They also engage in a funny kind of dance called, of all things, "crown shyness."

Crown, or in Latin, as fate would have it, *corona*.

Perhaps you've seen this yourself: tree canopies that create elaborate green puzzles of almost-touching crowns. Looking up, each branch of green is haloed by sky, creating a sort of cerebellum patchwork. There are different theories about why trees do this—to nourish the young plants below, to maximize resource sharing and reduce competition, to let the light through. But in any case, the limbs and branches maintain a safe distance for the benefit of the whole ecosystem, even as the roots embrace, invisibly, beneath the surface.

Years on, crown shyness still feels like a life-giving metaphor for times of rest or convalescence. If our nervous systems or our immune function demand apparent separation, you might not see us out in the world. But beneath the surface, we are very much part of the whole living web. Even as our limbs sway separately, spaciously, our roots are deep and intertwined—connecting invisibly below, showing us that we're in this together.

In this final verse of our embodied writing practice, we're putting all the pieces together. Noticing the ways in which we are fundamentally supported, alive, and accompanied. We're learning to lean into this wider web of support, whether in nature, the human community, or spirit. What might it look like to attend to the circulation of resource in a larger sense? To trust our deep-rooted connection to the larger forest?

As always, this isn't a thought exercise but a deeply bodied practice that considers how we live as well as we can with the conditions, histories, and sensitivities we have. Caring for and keeping our embodied writing practice will help guide the way.

Practice

GATHERING IN AWE

On April 8, 2024, a total eclipse passed through western Maine. In the weeks leading up to the event, everyone seemed to be in anticipation. By way of greeting, people would ask each other about their eclipse plans. *You gonna watch? Did you order your glasses?* When the day finally arrived, it was indeed a celestial magic that was out of this world, of a magnitude I'm still trying to comprehend. But what really got me was something supremely human: *We gathered in awe.* We came together with strangers because wonder and beauty and cosmic amazement compelled us to do so.

Which, at this moment on the planet, is rare. We tend to coalesce in groups and subgroups, political groups, affiliations, parent groups. Consider your own calendar with its doctor's appointments or meetings, friends and family, sports events, support groups. In all these configurations, we're loosely bound by *a thing we're trying to do or people we have something in common with.*

But it wasn't task or denomination that compelled us out to Rangeley, Maine, to sit ourselves on the long slope of a south-facing hill. We packed snacks and chairs, brought the dog, because who knew what the traffic would be on the way home (significant, it turned out). We went without much of a plan, part of a great happening that we didn't understand but were game to try.

When the moment arrived, and the black orb of the moon passed in front of the sun, no one on that hillside was immune to the magnificence. There were cries of beauty and surprise, stunned exclamations of "Can you believe this?!" Even Nora, my teenager, for whom idling on a hillside was not a relished activity, lit in delight when the sky turned blue-black and the frozen lake below became something else entirely. As the golden warmth of sunlight returned, applause broke out over the crowd. Listening to the radio on the way home, we heard children and reporters alike giddy, awash in feeling for all of it: the silver ring of light, the wild temperature swings, our place in the sky.

I don't tend to throw in with strangers. As a craniosacral therapist, I'm less likely to tailgate than launch into a screed on the dangers of traumatic brain injuries. But wonder as an organizing force? An experience to behold rather than debate? This I can get behind.

We cannot orchestrate celestial events; these wild happenings are singular and fleeting. But for days, I buzzed. Gathering there, all of us in awe together, lit something wordless and wonderful that I couldn't see until the darkness came.

Engage the Body

In this practice we return to one of our essential ingredients in embodied writing: Reverence. Pure, unadulterated, noncorrective gazing that simply says *wow*.

Imagine a gathering organized around wonder. What happens in your body when you think of a collective field that requires no talking, doing, or deciding? Perhaps you notice a wider breath, an invisible smile?

Now imagine you might create a gathering that distills this essence, a fantasy celebration you can visit in your mind's eye. A bit like an *oh wow* party or a gathering in awe. There will be no effort on your part, no small talk, no lingering beyond your timeline, no compromises of body or energy. This may be a gathering of only you. Just a tableau of wonder you're creating to visit whenever you like.

Write

First, grab your notebook, and start dreaming: Think of a place or image that fills you with wonder. A waterfall. A wide-open prairie. The city at twilight. Then, how will you linger in wonder? Are there picnic blankets, pool floats, magical golden bubbles? (This is your party and your fantasy—anything goes!) Is there food? Music? What else companions you in this space? Animals, sunshine, other people, wild turkeys, vast emptiness—be extravagant in your imagining.

Practice
BEAUTY

Beauty can be an internal and even invisible experience, one that teaches us to reclaim a loveliness that only we may recognize. Sometimes, an experience of beauty—a glint of light on water, the deep fuchsia of a dahlia's petal, or the bend in a river—can interrupt our painful stories and bring us to a present moment imbued with grace. Noticing where we find beauty can create a kind of compass of the heart, guiding our attention toward what moves us and waking us up to the right now.

The poetry of haiku is spare, open, and direct—a wonderful blueprint for beauty. Forget the rules about syllables you learned in primary school and instead lean into writer Natalie Goldberg's description:

> What is the Way of haiku? Bare attention, no distractions, pure awareness, noticing only what is in the moment. Being connected to seasons, unconnected to self-clinging. And then, out of that, composing your experience in three lines that go beyond logic, that make the mind leap. In the center, a taste of emptiness. A frog, a crow, a turnip—the ordinary right in front of you is the realm of awakening. Pure Zen but not Zen.[21]

There are so many wonderful examples of haiku—an invitation to explore haiku on your own, particularly from masters of the craft, like Issa, Basho, and Buson. As you do, see if you can feel that "taste of emptiness" Goldberg names. Notice how nimble and present these quiet lines are, how unbound by story or logic.

Write

Borrowing Goldberg's "three lines that go beyond logic, that make the mind leap," let your body be still and your mind nimble. Then, noticing beauty within and around you, play with creating your own haiku.

Deepen

After you've written a few of your own haiku, read them aloud (to yourself or a pet or a plant or the room). As you read, see if you can let your perception include your bodied sensations as you attend to beauty. How does this experience change or stretch your notions of beauty? What does beauty feel like here?

SISTER ROSIE

On a winter evening, I gathered with my friends Molly and Colleen in the studio behind Molly's house. We'd closed the doors and sat together on the couch, talking and snacking on blueberries and chocolate. As they always do, our conversations went deep and wide, traversing the aches and celebrations of motherhood, middle age, protest, art. But we weren't here to only talk, and after a while Colleen said, "Well, should we play some music?"

We plugged in a guitar and bass, reached for our lyrics, and sang. PJ Harvey and Lucinda Williams covers, a rocking ballad Molly wrote for Gemma, her deceased chicken.

Never mind the chaos around us: Molly's sewing machines and piles of fabric for her work as a seamstress. Small flats full of sprouting seeds. Never mind the chaos outside: a child clamoring at the window, shouting, "Mom! Where are the pretzels?"

Because here, in our circle of voices and instruments, something else was happening. A kind of magic. Our little band, Sister Rosie, doesn't perform, record, or promote; we play for the pure joy of being together like this.

I'm sure humans make something better than music, but I can't think of what that is.

How singing has wound its way through your life can be its own kind of biography. Were there lullabies? Were you raised around voices that sang? Did you hear your grandmother in the choir?

In my childhood, music was ever present. My sisters and I sang while we waited at the bus stop; we paused in our sibling fights to harmonize a song and then got back to hitting each other. We sang around the table in Sweden, carefully studying the words to every dirty drinking song. Of which there were many. On St. Lucia Day in December, we'd be recruited to join my mother's group of Swedish expats to sing angelically as hot candle wax dripped on our heads and hands.

Someone once asked me how love was expressed in my origin family, and I flapped silently, like a fish. "It—well, we—they . . ." I ran through a reel of family memories and saw no evidence of North American love, the kind marked by frequent "I love yous," compliments, and embrace. But what shall we call this feeling of being wrapped in music and stories? Of this abundant, inclusive cacophony that joins you in collective exaltation? Music was its own love language, a place where voice and body could meet and move.

Like writing, my relationship to singing started easy and natural and then became tight and compressed when I held it up for evaluation. For a time, I became music adjacent, mooning over my friends' talents, awestruck as they played. If a guitar came out around a campfire, I stayed quiet, secretly wishing to play. In later adulthood, making music again brought parts of myself back online. Parts that would prove essential in the depths of illness.

When my autoimmune disease was flaring, I'd fill the bathtub and sit in the dark, singing a melody from some deep place. When things got so bad that voice itself felt unreachable, Molly and Colleen came over and offered the only thing that calmed my body and mind. They sank with me, lower and lower, down to the ground, until we cradled our guitars, leaned sideways on our elbows. With them nearby, I could pluck a string, hum. We found a chord progression, two words, and enough strength to strum.

Just this, we sang. Calling ourselves back in.

Practice

SING

In this practice, we're exploring music and song as a gesture of love. We'll use humming to loosen up and find new expressions, making space for a different kind of medicine.

Engage the Body

Without planning, preparation, words, or music, begin to hum. Follow whatever melody emerges, getting curious about the lilt and rhythm, the feeling that arises organically.

Place a hand on your chest and lips to feel the vibration of this sound.

Perhaps there are words that want to be sung? Memories? Wishes? Do your hands want to clap a rhythm to your melody? Does a familiar song rise to the surface?

Write

Pause and consider how music and song are woven through your life. *A memory of music . . .*

Deepen

Tenderly bring to mind an earlier version of you, one in need of comfort or inclusion. With hands resting on heart and belly, offer this part a lullaby that you make up on the spot, remember, or simply hum.

FIRST PERSON

Becoming Body Forward

Marcella is a mom who's loved and lost an angel child. Here she explores listening through her body as a means to reconnect to life and tell the story of the child she lost.

As a young mother, I received the devastating news that my daughter, Ruthie, would likely not live beyond the age of eight. A neurodegenerative process was ravaging her brain and body. Dementia in a child. Exact dosing of medications, dietary restrictions, endless evaluations, ICU stays, biopsies, constant seizure and pica precautions. (Pica is the condition of eating nonfood items.) For years I lived a life of precision. There was no night or day or weekends off from the medical management, even when she was in hospital care. A slight mistake could mean the onset of acute illness or even death. Ruthie lived ten more birthdays beyond the predicted eight. She passed from her earthly body to an angel form when she was eighteen. I stayed behind to continue raising her three very active and healthy younger brothers.

In and around my on-call nurse mom role, I experienced other significant losses. My parents, my greatest support system, died a month apart. My best friend, the library of my life, died from cancer. My marriage died too, and with that I lost my home, community, and eventually even my health insurance. I suffered two freak falls, resulting in a broken body with varying degrees of pain and metal replacement parts that don't function or feel like the original parts. These losses also required a lot of brain power to maintain some sort of sanity. I missed the me who loved speed, travel, nature, laughing, a starry sky, live concerts, dancing, making fires, and the comfort of my amazing friends. But how could I actually return to feeling better? How could I achieve my desire to tell Ruth's story?

Several years ago, through the guidance, patience, and love of the author of this book, I began to work on a different approach to living my life. I began to start my days with a check-in of my physical body, along with my heart and soul, before allowing the brain power to take over. I asked my body how it would feel most comfortable in the day ahead. How could I provide the comfort, safety, and care it deserved? It has taken practice, but it has opened new paths I hadn't seen at the beginning and steadily brought me back to myself.

Today I am free from the brain chains as much as life will allow. The nervous system has calmed. The practice of living more fully in my body even allows me to reflect on the past in a different way. Instead of the linear timeline of traumatic medical events and challenges, I focus on the gifts, joy, and tremendous courage in it all. I live in gratitude for my life and the imperfect body I live it in. I am able to use embodied writing to finally create the memoir about my angel child. Ruth's story does not need the brain precision. Her story is in the pure love of living life with a terminal child. And all the feelings—the pain, the joy, the frustrations, sorrow, and even the humor. When I look up at the night sky, or watch the clouds roll by whenever I fly, I can feel my sweet Ruthie in the warmth of my heart, and I smile.

Practice

MOVEMENTS

At my wedding, I watched my cousin—lanky, towering, and fine boned—step onto a dance floor for the first time. She looked around at the others twisting and turning to the music, and . . . started jumping. Feet together, arms at her side, she sailed above the crowd in great, unstoppable, pogo-stick bounds. She danced like this for hours, her face beaming in discovery and arrival. She seemed to respond to a call to *just move.*

My cousin was showing us that when the music compels you, *go*. We need not wait until we figure it out before we act. If we are committed to movement, we need to *move*. And rarely are new movements graceful. They are bumbling and unfamiliar and create something new.

Here in our practice, let us acknowledge the power of movements. Movements that join us collectively, movements that compel us individually, movements that are neither graceful nor practiced but respond to a deeper pull; movements that create something we haven't seen before.

Engage the Body

Perhaps putting on a song you love or simply allowing your own body to tell you how it wants to stretch, let yourself move.

Write

I am moved by . . .

Practice

HIPS

When you hear the word *posture*, do you quietly rake your shoulders back and extend your neck? Do you suddenly lose awareness of your legs and stop breathing?

Somewhere along the way, posture became synonymous with "sit up straight." We lost the true meaning of the word, "a state of being in relation to circumstances." At its roots, posture isn't about rigidity but connection. How we move in relationship to the whole.

Your pelvis and hips are your postural foundation, a meeting place between lower and upper parts of the body. You might even rock a little bit in the pelvis and see if you can trace how this movement echoes up in your shoulders and neck and down into the legs. This anatomical bowl is also an important house of organ systems, including digestion, elimination, and sex. Of course, it's also essential to dance.

This area also houses one of my favorite bones, the sacrum. This lovely triangle at the very base of the spine is a bit like your own personal throne. A sacred seat for only you. The word *craniosacral* conveys the intimate connection between the cranio (from cranium, your skull) and the sacral (sacrum). These areas are intimately connected through various anatomical, fluid, and energetic channels. Craniosacral therapists like to say: "as above, so below." Which is another way of saying that the fluidity we welcome into the hips reverberates everywhere else.

As you explore the hips, you might consider some of these questions that speak to posture in the sense of connection: What does coherence and connection feel like for me? How do I move through transitions? How might I water the seeds of my own creative practice? How do I foster real connections, within my own body, the natural world, and with other humans?

One of the gifts of this anatomical bowl is that it has space for a lot of reimagining. We can listen in the key of creativity, reclaiming posture not as rigidity but possibility.

Engage the Body

Placing your hands on your hips, invite some soft rocking: forward and back, side to side, rotations. Widen your awareness to see if you can notice how this central point connects to feet, to ribs, to shoulders.

Then, from lying down or sitting, move into a figure-four stretch: Cross your left ankle over your right thigh and interlace your fingers behind your right thigh. Next you can either gently pull in toward your chest or lean forward, deepening into the hips. Repeat on the opposite side.

Write

Taking inspiration from Lucille Clifton's extraordinary poem, "Homage to My Hips," write into the prompt *These hips need . . .*

Deepen

Whether you're lying down, sitting up, or cooking in the kitchen, play some music that encourages your hips to move.

THE SAGES IN THE ATTIC

2017. The sound of giggling was loud up in the attic. Nora and her best friend had decided they were a band—Family Freeze Dance, they called themselves—and were using an old cassette player to record their frenetic, squealing, strumming, yelling, talking "music." A peek behind the door revealed a vision of summertime seven-year-olds: covered in bug bites and dirt, missing teeth, routinely distracted by fart jokes.

But there was another kind of magic happening up there too, one that we sometimes forget on our way to adulthood: Delight in communion. Resonant joy. No one was managing the other's experience, worrying over how they are, or trying to help.

I'm thinking about this as I remember a conversation with a client on what it means to be responsible. Many of us, many of us women in particular, have grown up with the sense that we need to track and manage the well-being of everyone in our orbit. To take on what they're feeling. To make it okay. Those expectations come early, with an insidious subtlety.

But follow that a little further and we can end up coming to all kinds of bizarre conclusions: That things will fall apart without our help, that we need to catch anyone around us who falls. That if we aren't caretaking, we'll be left.

Our good intentions unwittingly say something else. Because if everyone needs helping, no one's quite right as they are.

Of course, we *do* need each other. Lots and lots. But if you'll allow me a little semantic latitude, *taking care with* each other is different from *caretaking* each other. We want the people we care for to feel better, but we cannot do the feeling for them. We are neither responsible for that nor entitled to it.

In part V we explored the fullness of our ecosystems and what it might feel like to show up without fixing. But now, with these seven-year-olds leading the way, we can go further, imagining spaces not just of witness but play. Spaces where we practice co-creation, the sublime experience of being enveloped in our own making while feeling held and connected. Of course, practicing embodied writing in group settings (more on how to do this on page 245) is a form of co-creation, but it can look all kinds of ways. Bird-watching. Band practice. Cooking. The spaces may be virtual or asynchronous depending on what our bodies need. The point is a communion that lets us show up with creative fullness.

Years later, I can see something else those kids upstairs with their very, very loud "music" were showing us: We are here to remind each other of who we already are. Creating together is one of the most elegant ways to return to the unhindered selves that have always been here, beneath it all. We may support that process for each other, but in important ways, we don't do anything except show up.

Which is everything.

RETREAT VS. REFUGE

"After a while Sophia asked, 'Are you sure the door is closed?'
'It's open,' her grandmother said. 'It's always open; you can sleep quite easy.'"

—*Tove Jansson,* The Summer Book[22]

I confess there have been moments, in the overwhelm of life, when I have wished for a cave. A quiet retreat that blocked out the noise of the world.

If I could just have a bit of quiet stillness, I'd think, *an unreachable cave where my only job was to sit in the dark, then I'd really be able to rest and reset.* Who among us has not craved an escape like this at one point or another?

But then, visiting family and bumping around Colorado, I went to an actual cave. One with dark chambers and stalactites hanging from the ceilings and strange, otherworldly mineral formations (also, tour guides and a gift shop just outside).

It was thrilling to walk and crawl through the place, but it turns out a cave may not be the solution I was looking for. As an introvert with chronic illness, it's not infrequent for me to crave a retreat, but what actually sustains me is refuge.

The distinction between retreat and refuge feels important for tender-hearted folks to explore, lest we accidentally walk around thinking that in order to receive real care we need to drop out of life.

Retreat is a place to get away to: a cabin on the mountain, a spa, a cave. Imagine thick walls and no interference, away from the requirements of life. If you've experienced a getaway like this, you know it can be a divine and fragile peace. It is, by nature, fleeting. You've left regular life to receive its benefits, but regular life still waits outside the door. This is maybe one of the (many) shortcomings of the notion of self-care; it's an individual pause that does nothing to change actual structures of care or make living more sustainable. But I digress.

I think of refuge as a tent with the flaps open: The breeze comes through, there's dirt on the floor, we can hear the sounds of life, just outside. Through refuge, we create shelter in the midst of messy life. It's an ongoing practice of residing in the self that does not bury or bypass our pain, grief, or loneliness; that doesn't wait for perfect conditions to return to ourselves.

Both retreat and refuge have their gifts, and from the outside they may look utterly indistinguishable. One December, when I pulled off the quadruple crown of flu, COVID, minor surgery, and invasive procedure, I absolutely retreated, closed the tent flaps, and turned out the lights. But once I was out of the acute phase, I could feel the pulse of something larger. I still needed deep rest, but I didn't need to be quite so closed off.

And closed off is where retreat becomes airless. Because if we draw back from every conversation / situation /experience that isn't comfortable, or wait endlessly for circumstances to be exactly right, we miss opportunities for real transformation and growth. We stop listening for how regular life might be more breathable (asterisk here: in times of overwhelm or danger, retreat may be precisely what we need, and the best choice available).

How we cultivate refuge can be a rich exploration. After I visited the desert, sea-level felt like refuge. Also daily writing, honest conversations, the warm mug of tea in my hands. And if this sounds a bit like locating what resources us without bypassing or denying our aches? Yes, exactly.

A final anecdote to hold in your pocket: I once heard a parable of a meditation retreat at which a large construction project outside was making all kinds of noise. "Ugh!" cried the meditators, "how are we supposed to cultivate calm with all that racket?" To which the teacher replied, "What do you think I pay them for?"

Practice

CULTIVATING REFUGE

Cultivating refuge amid the larger world can change our relationship to repair and convalescence. We're no longer perched in anticipation of when it all gets better; we're listening in the here and now for ease.

When I asked our embodied writing online community what helps them locate refuge in their own lives, they returned with a trove of riches:

The new neighborhood we're moving to. Potlucks. Watering my garden. My art. A breeze on my face. Soil in my hands. Dancing so completely that everyone disappears. When I can sit quietly and observe my husband connecting with our kids. Can refuge be a verb? I am refuging now, something like that. Prayer. Full permission to be as silly or as quiet as I feel in that moment. Definitely a nap. Community. The moments when I have just completed a task or job and am able to take a beat to feel content. A hot bath and maybe a "corny" Reader's Digest *that a neighbor gave me. A conversation that takes a vulnerable shift down to the heart. Hanging the laundry on the line and taking a full breath. Always a walk alone in the woods. A quiet corner to eat my sandwich.*

Engage the Body

Now it's your turn, friends. Creating as much comfort in your body as possible, bring refuge to mind.

Write

What helps you locate refuge in your own life?

Practice

GIMME SHELTER

Back when Nora was three or four years old, we were playing outside in the snow one day and decided to build a house.

"What does a house need?" I asked.

"Well," she said thoughtfully, "A toilet. And some art. Oh, and a kitchen!"

It did feel like a very complete list.

As we explore refuge, we can follow Nora's lead and bring real play to the inquiry of *what houses us.* Our shelters might include not only literal buildings, but routines, rituals, favorite slippers, verdant gardens, and particular practices.

We might get poetic with our whole notion of a nervous system, imagining a kind of beautiful exoskeleton that moves with us, fed by living structures of support that offer us respite amid the messy and imperfect.

Engage the Body

Letting your notion of shelter be both wide and soft, see what comes to your awareness as you consider the structures you inhabit.

Write

I am housed by . . .

Deepen

Structure describes a wide range of matter. It could be a rigid and heavy railroad bridge, a chain-link fence beside a highway, or the supple spines of a sea anemone. Slowing down offers important information on how structures feel to us from within: Is this a place we want to linger? Get close to? Escape?

Explore these short sprint prompts and notice what comes up as you write into each of these words for a minute or two:

- Rock wall
- Honeycomb
- Chambers of the heart
- Jungle gym
- Fire escape

Practice

FRAGILE BUT REGENERATIVE: THINKING IN SEASONS

One winter morning when my heart was heavy with news of the world, I took our dog Rosie on a walk that followed the path behind the dump. We skirted the edges of the snowless marsh, following the trail down through the trees. In the small ruts of frozen mud were filaments of ice, thin membranes that crackled under her paws and my boots. Fragile, I realized, but if I widened my attention beyond the right now, also regenerative.

Because in spring this spot would turn soft and thick until the green came, receding cold to memory. In fall the path would be covered in leaves. Budding and blooming, fading and dying. Our bodies do the same. We bleed. We breathe. The chambers of the heart contract and release. We shed and regrow. Life pulses in and through regardless. Thinking in cycles and longer timelines felt like a kinder frame, one that could help us discern seasons of searching and connecting, resting and seeding. Individually and collectively, we're always moving through something.

The red dog did not wait for me in my reverie. She'd already gone ahead, exploring the bramble, crunching patches of ice along the way.

Practice

From the beginning, our work has been to become intimate with what resources us and to discern beneath the surface—even in those moments when we feel broken or stuck—our own aliveness. In this practice we're bringing the lens of seasons to regard the greater unfolding in our lives.

Consider these distinct gestures: summer's abundance, fall's fading and letting go, winter's stillness, spring's beginning again.

Writing

Inviting yourself to be generous and kind as you regard your own life, grab your notebook and explore: *What have been your summers, autumns, winters, and springs?*

Practice

DREAMING

I once dreamed of a giant herd of bulls running underwater. Looking down from above I was both awed and frightened by their massive, powerful forms.

It can be so tempting to decipher what a dream means, to rush to decode some hidden message. Instead, I prefer slowing down to explore the imagery, to let the dreams keep speaking. This pause in our rush to make meaning opens a dialogue with that essentially mysterious place within us.

Regardless of how you dream, our exploration here is about lingering in the rich terrain of dream imagery. And because dreams are, well, dreamy, we'll be a little more experimental with our explorations.

Engage the Body

For this exercise, bring to mind an image or scene from a compelling dream. If nothing comes to mind, feel free to imagine something dreamlike.

Next, gather your pens and paper (and colored pencils or paints if you choose) and gently ask your inner censor to step away. As Austrian poet Rainer Maria Rilke writes, "You must give birth to your images. They are the future waiting to be born." There is potency in our dream images.

Draw

Take your time drawing this dream image. Let yourself be surprised by whatever emerges.

Deepen

Staying with this image, write into what you see. Rather than creating a coherent narrative, play with descriptions, movements, emotion, colors, pairs of opposites, shapes and gestures. Perhaps there's a poem hidden in this dream image?

Practice
FLEDGING

fledged; fledging intransitive verb
of a young bird: to acquire the feathers necessary for flight or independent activity
also : to leave the nest after acquiring such feathers

Since Nora was two we've kept a small flock of chickens in a coop out by the garden. Every few springs we order a new batch of chicks from the Farmer's Union. The birds start out fuzzy and cute, cheeping together under a heat lamp in the basement, become strange and awkward pullets with stray feathers and long necks, and eventually, as they fluff up and the crate begins to feel too small, we transition them to join the older flock in the big coop. We've watched this cycle play out over years, a reliable move from growing to *out*growing.

In an old video, Nora's toddler body lumbers after the birds, opening her arms and calling out, "Hang on! Hang on!" Her movements are adorably bumbling; she wants so much to corral those chickens that her voice buzzes with excitement. If only they would just hold up a minute and wait for her.

That toddler is now a teenager, and in a few years she'll move on from this phase too. The speed takes my breath away. Wasn't I just admiring her baby fingers? Watching her jump off the porch, plastic bags held aloft, trying to fly? Some part of me is skipping along after her, flailing my arms, crying, "Hang on! Hang on!" Couldn't she possibly slow down?

But of course, she cannot.

Despite my tender heart, letting go for the next chapter is part of the parental job description. Fledging is essential to flight. If we are alive and growing, we will bust out of the earlier versions of our life, we will expand our capacity and our range. We'll reach a point when the nest will no longer do. It's as true for birds as it is for humans.

Here in our explorations through embodied writing, we arrive at the necessary ache of letting go of what we've outgrown. Learning to live well in the bodies we have will never be a rule-following enterprise or a static set of guidelines. Instead, we notice what no longer fits us and make room for movement and change.

And then, if we are lucky, there will be moments—tender, unsteady, but supported—when we stretch a little further, summon as best we can a trust in these new feathers, and ready ourselves for flight.

Not if we're chickens, though. Then we just run around making a lot of noise.

Engage the Body

In part I, we explored coming into present time to notice if there were any micro-adjustments that might create less constriction. Here we'll expand this inquiry further, making way for adjustments in the larger field.

Begin by dropping your attention into your body. Are there areas that feel too tight or crowded?

Take a moment to tune toward these places and adjust accordingly. Perhaps a belt, a breath, or a hair tie might like to be a little looser.

Now widen your attention to include the space around you, letting your eyes roam the room. Do you notice anything that feels dusty or limiting? Brittle or stuck?

Now explore even further afield, flying through various parts of your life. What wants more spaciousness?

Write

Find your notebook and write into *What is ready to let go? What is ready to take flight?*

A HOSPITAL IS NOT A QUIET PLACE

Sunlight was finally shining on the hospital windows and lighting up the snow of yesterday's storm, casting Portland in a brilliance I did not feel. In those last days of 2019 I was hoping next year might be a turn for the better, not knowing how supremely, globally wrong that would be. Jon sat by my bed. He had come bearing a trove of kindnesses to make this place more bearable: books and comfortable clothes, salt, pepper, lemon, and butter to add flavor to the hospital food.

Around us, the hospital was a busy, bustling, peopled place. Nurses, doctors, techs, phlebotomists, specialists of all stripes, pharmacists. I wondered how a building designed to house and cure could run so counter to any notion of rest. My roommate's bed alarm went off at all hours, my IV unit ran out of fluid and began screeching, the woman next door shouted that she *HAS TO GET OUT OF HERE! WHO CAN HELP HER? WHO?* Clicking, popping beeping, crashing, time passage marked by checks of vital signs, the movement of light across the room, the wait for the doctor, always the wait, and then finally arriving flanked by students, forming a sudden amphitheater around you.

Did you know you would be performing this morning in a one-act play about your colon?

There was relief that the pretense of managing any of this was gone. There were drugs, good, strong drugs, that eased the wince frozen across my face. And new tiles to study. I had spent so much time in the bathroom—on the floor, passed out on the toilet, sobbing in the shower, struggling with childproof caps—that I had a strange fascination with these ones, small beige tiles set off with flecks of white. I spent time arranging the patterns in my mind, staring at my pale-blue hospital-issue socks, both sides printed with tacky nonskid plastic. Impossible to tell which side was up.

The last time I was hospitalized I'd kept the admission secret, telling myself that the weight of anyone else's worry would be too much to bear. And so I'd created this small invisible tent, just me and Jon inside while the rest of the world hummed along. *You didn't even tell your parents?* a friend asked, incredulously. *What kind of crazy person would isolate herself at the moment she most needed help?* A crazy person who had made the calculation: easier to just deal with myself, thanks.

Perhaps I didn't want to cop to being a sick person with overwhelming needs. I told myself I was protecting them from worry, but the truth, closer in, was that I feared they wouldn't be there, and so didn't give them a chance to show up. I'd believed that walling myself off from sympathy would temper the chaos and fragility. But now I understood how wrong that was. Hiding my pain and pretending I needed nothing wasn't a kindness but a brutal, isolating fiction.

This time, drained of pretense, I leaned on them. Pilar drove me to the infusion center for an IV of fluids. Molly and Colleen came over to play music and lay on the floor beside me, strumming and singing. Many meals were delivered. My sister Melina sent me packages of new soft underwear. My desperately worried mother called every day, the relief at being in touch audible in her voice.

It was startling to name the thing I wanted. More startling to have it heard. Instead of holding the world at arm's length, I collapsed into it, becoming porous and softer.

One morning, in a haze of medication and sleeplessness, I had a kind of waking dream. I was borne on the back of a giant bird, and we swooped and flew through different scenes of my life. Meredith and me in a kitchen in Costa Rica, doubled over in laughter after another pressure cooker mishap, garbanzo beans covering every surface. Walking down Walden Street to the corner spa—Bostonian for bodega—with Molly and Hannah and Alyssa, eating Twizzlers, spilling the tea. Here were kind strangers, younger cousins, my grandmother. We banked and flew over sweet encounters at bus stops, summer camps, infusion rooms. Charlie dog, walking beside me through the woods with his quiet dignity and watchfulness. Connections, everywhere. Onward, until I was back in the hospital room, Jon holding my hand, Nora curled beside me in the bed.

My reverie was broken by a bed alarm and a loud voice that suddenly called out from across the room.

"Hey!" My roommate directed her comments not at me but Jon. "Your wife really knows how to advocate for herself, did you know that?"

I hadn't thought of it that way, but she wasn't wrong. When the nurse declared my pain was resolving, I'd simply said that it was not. When the doctor delivered an alarmist, blaming screed ("The Crohn's patient on the seventh floor is doing better, but for some reason you're not"), I'd explained I needed time to think about what she'd said. I wasn't doing anything special. I'd listened to their expertise. I just hadn't ignored my own. Unbeknownst to me, I'd had this witness the whole time.

"Yeah," my roommate went on. "I've never seen anyone do it like that. She's kind, but she's not getting pushed around in here."

Not getting pushed around in here. Somewhere along the way, something had shifted. I'd felt so brittle and walled off in the early days of my disease. Convinced I had to maintain the appearance of health rather than discovering what health could mean. I didn't know how to listen to my body or what it needed, didn't have tools for knowing myself from the inside, and I certainly didn't have language or the temerity to share how I honestly felt. It took years for that old veneer to crumble. My hospital mate helped me see what I'd be cultivating, the jewels of which you are holding in your hands right now.

"Safety is not the absence of a threat, it is the presence of connection," writes physician and author Gabor Maté. Even if I was skeletal, disarranged, and hopeless, this was also true: I wasn't alone in all this. This writing, this body, and this practice had made me looser and more breathable. They helped me develop both a spine that trusted my knowing, a widening softness for the world, and a voice unafraid to name it. The hallmark of all real healing is not the transformation into someone new, but the reclamation of what we've been all along. Love had risen to meet me, a miracle every time.

Practice

NUMINOUS

In this practice we're preparing the field for the numinous: encounters with grace-filled awe. For me, these meetings have nothing to do with denomination or belief; they aren't even necessarily special. Instead, they arrive by way of a looking that's willing to be moved by what it sees. It's a kind of attention that's awake to the mysterious splendor of the world.

I've felt numinousness in the sounds of an oboe. The way rain collects in perfect spheres on the leaves of a lupine. A poem so beautifully rendered and timed that it unraveled something. In these moments, the canvas widens. I remember that life pulses through every part.

Engage the Body

Bring to mind a moment when your experience of the world bloomed in new awareness. This could be something quiet and unexceptional that didn't register as extraordinary to anyone else but ignited in you a sense of the largeness of life. A firefly. A hummingbird. A piece of music drifting from an open window.

Holding this memory, imagine a horizon stretching out before you in all directions. Let your body orient to the spaciousness of these long sight lines. Then feel your midline descending through your spine and also up toward the sky. In this vastness, let your attention rest in your pulsing heart.

Write

We are made of . . .

Practice

ARE YOU HEALED NOW?

As we arrived at the end of our session, I noticed Ellie shifting in her chair.

"Johanna, can I ask you something?"

"Yes, of course," I said.

"So you've lived with chronic illness for a long time, right?" She paused. It felt like we were leaning in close to something. "Are you . . . healed?"

These tender questions matter; if we don't rush through them they're often pointing inward, leading us toward an important truth. Ellie was naming what I think we're all secretly wondering: *Did you figure it out? Can I? Is there hope even for me?*

"I used to believe," I said, "that *healed* was a final destination, a turnstile I could pass through, clap my hands together and declare, 'Whew! Thank God that's over.' But that hasn't been my actual experience."

I told her about the long process of writing this book. How in the early days, it was a story about getting sick and getting better and then, when I got really sick again in 2019, I thought the book was ruined. *So much for a story of healing.*

But it turned out that *healed* didn't have to be a flimsy, conditional state, where every symptom is a failure exiling you back to the land of the diseased. Instead, healing started to feel like an inquiry, one that pulled me toward a new set of questions: What does it mean to be a true friend to yourself? How do you live well in the body you have? How can writing and embodiment feed your unfolding life?

These days it feels more interesting and kinder to practice this inner allegiance that doesn't turn on whether I'm sick or healed but lets me be more honest about what's happening inside, which in turn lets me live among the messy world.

"So I guess," I said, "I'm not healed in terms of free of symptoms. Not free of despair, not free of wishing this would all quiet down already. But definitely freer, and that makes me feel healthier than I've ever been." She knew what it meant to live through her own deep losses and traumas but perhaps didn't know that these questions and conversations were medicine for me too. Meeting in these tender places to move and write and share is some of the best healing I know.

Engage the Body

Relaxing into the embodied writing practice you've been cultivating over these pages, consider what healing means from here. Are you healed? What might you offer yourself or someone else about what healing means?

Write

Healing looks like . . .

Deepen

Poets from Thomas Merton to Andrea Gibson to Joy Harjo write in praise of wholeness as a truth granted to every being, a truth worth celebrating and exploring. See if you can take a few breaths to sense into the wholeness of your own being. How might you imagine this feeling? As an orb of light around you? A calm surface of water, clear and bright? What might you offer yourself to tend to this invisible wholeness? (Remember that revisiting your list of *what feels good* to add lavishly to whatever resources you is always an option!)

Practice

RIPENING AND LETTING GO

The end of a workshop series feels a bit like late summer. We've prepared the soil, planted seeds, watched them grow, and now we are into harvest season. Tomatoes ripe and juicy, watermelons full on the vine. Late summer is such a distinct time that even the word *harvest* comes from the old English *hærfest*: the period between August and October. In some traditions late summer is its own fifth season. This is a season of resting in the ripeness that precedes letting go.

It is also the season of curing. Not curing as in free from all suffering, but curing as in brined and flavorful, bright and crisp. Gardeners distill what they've harvested to an essence that will last through all seasons by preserving the bounty: Garlic hangs from the rafters, cucumbers become pickles in brine.

And it is here in our work together, after we have moved and written, shared, shed layers, discovered new language, relished in communion, that I like to share one of my favorite poems, "Da Capo," by Jane Hirshfield (the ending lines of which you'll find at the very beginning of this book). In the poem, Hirshfield brings the reader into the body, gathering, preparing, cooking, and then tasting until gifting us these final lines:

You may do this, I tell you, it is permitted.
Begin again the story of your life.

Here at the end of the poem, we begin again—the title itself, "Da Capo," is a musical note meaning *from the top*. And here, at the end of our practice, we also begin again. Trusting that the cycle continues.

Engage the Body

Either lying down or sitting, bring your body into stillness. Then move sequentially through your body from feet to head: tightening/gripping each part on an inhale and then releasing on an exhale. Include legs, torso, hands, arms, shoulders, face. Finally, tighten and release all the muscles in the body. Rest for a few moments to notice how you feel.

Write

You may do this, I tell you, it is permitted . . .

Deepen

Consider your harvests and harvest seasons; consider the softening you've done over these pages. What might it mean to *begin again the story of your life?* What new permission do you have in the telling? What reverence might you bring to your own unfolding life?

PRACTICING EMBODIED WRITING WITH OTHERS

Whether you're practicing with a partner or a group, embodied writing can deepen meaningfully when enjoyed with others. It's remarkable what happens in a setting imbued with permission, reverence, kind witness, and reflection. Embodied writing groups have birthed deep friendships, supportive connections, and long-term writing partnerships. If you'd like to practice with someone else, here are some steps to get started:

Invite. As you consider who to practice with, let folks know that this will be a gathering of movement and mutual support rather than writing critique. Encourage participants to read through part I, "Orientation," to let them know what's involved.

Prepare the container. Once you've found a partner or group to practice with and settled on a location and date, encourage participants to be easy and loose, inviting them to dress comfortably, bring a notebook and pen or pencil, and perhaps tea or snacks to share (chocolate is always a good idea!)

Gather. Using the chapter "Setting the Foundations" in part I as a guide, begin with acknowledgments and a few minutes of settling and guided meditation or stillness. (On johannafranzel.com you can find links to audio meditations for settling.) Even if the members of your group know each other well, it's helpful to have a quick go-round to name a resource, an intention, and a quick (two sentence) check-in.

Remember. You have a body, and this is a space to honor that body. You are on this land in this season. Remember that our guiding principles are permission and reverence and that whatever is shared here will be held in confidence. (I like to mention these pieces at each gathering.)

Move. Choose a practice that speaks to you, read through the setup, and then take some time in movement, breath, or visualization. For practices that need props (tennis balls, blankets, foam rollers, etc.), make sure you have some handy.

Write. Share the writing prompt with the group, set a timer for ten minutes, and write. Encourage everyone to find a comfortable spot as they explore writing on their own.

Share. Even if it's a single word or sentence, consider speaking your words out loud. While reading what you've written is completely optional, it can also be a powerful experience to share your words out loud; doing so often reveals new discoveries, connections, or depth.

Reflect. It can be so tempting to analyze, praise, or discuss the pieces. Instead, simply repeat back a line or word that really moved you, letting the writer know how these words reverberate outward. You might find yourselves moving in surprising discussions.

Repeat! Begin again and repeat another practice or two, depending on the prompt.

Closing. Ending with a poem or a word or two that each person is taking with them can be a lovely way to bring closure to the gathering.

NOTES

1. Brenda Ueland, *If You Want to Write* (Graywolf Press, 1987), 29.
2. Saeed Jones, "I Believe in the Intelligence of Honey," *Werk-In-Progress*, Substack, October 2, 2019, https://open.substack.com/pub/saeedjones/p/coming-soon.
3. Susan Raffo, "Aligning the Relational Field: A Love Story About Retelling the Creation of Craniosacral Therapy (and a Lot of Other Touch-Based Therapy as Well)," January 25, 2020, https://www.susanraffo.com/blog/aligning-the-relational-field-a-love-story-about-retelling-the-creation-of-craniosacral-therapy-and-a-lot-of-other-touch-based-bodywork-as-well.
4. Albert Szent-Györgyi, "Biology and Pathology of Water," *Perspectives in Biology and Medicine*, John Hopkins University Press, Vol. 14, No. 2, Winter 1971: 239–249, https://doi.org/10.1353/pbm.1971.0014.
5. Melissa Febos, "Ode to an Outcast Part," in *The Book of Alchemy: A Creative Practice for an Inspired Life*, Suleika Jaouad, author (Random House, 2025), 169.
6. Florida Scott Maxwell, *The Measure of My Days: One Woman's Vivid, Enduring Celebration of Life and Aging* (Penguin Books, 1979).
7. Studs Terkel, "Studs Terkel in conversation with Sydney Lewis: Interviewing the World's Greatest Interviewer," interview by Sydney Lewis, Transom.org, August 1, 2001, https://transom.org/2001/studs-terkel-in-conversation/.
8. Ocean Vuong, "A Life Worth of Our Breath," interview by Krista Tippett, *On Being*, April 30, 2020, https://onbeing.org/programs/ocean-vuong-a-life-worthy-of-our-breath-2022/.
9. Darcy Banco, MD, MPH, Jerway Chang, MD, Nina Talmor, MD, et al. "Sex and Race Differences in the Evaluation and Treatment of Young Adults Presenting to the Emergency Department with Chest Pain," *Journal of the American Heart Association* (2022); Siobhan Fenton, "How Sexist Stereotypes

Mean Doctors Ignore Women's Pain," *The Independent*, July 27, 2016, https://www.the-independent.com/life-style/health-and-families/health-news/how-sexist-stereotypes-mean-doctors-ignore-women-s-pain-a7157931.html.

10. See, for example: Amy Roeder, "America Is Failing Its Black Mothers," *Harvard Public Health: Magazine of the Harvard T.H. Chan School of Public Health*, Winter 2019, accessed September 8, 2025, https://hsph.harvard.edu/news/america-is-failing-its-black-mothers/; Fred Clasen-Kelly, Renuka Rayasam, "Black Americans Still Suffer Worse Health. Here's Why There's So Little Progress," Shots Health News from NPR, October 24, 2024, accessed September 7, 2025, https://www.npr.org/sections/shots-health-news/2024/10/24/nx-s1-5162440/black-american-south-health-disparities-medicaid.
11. Sonya Huber, *Pain Woman Takes Your Keys, and Other Essays from a Nervous System* (University of Nebraska Press, 2017).
12. Huber, *Pain Woman.*
13. Suleika Jaouad, *The Book of Alchemy: A Creative Practice for an Inspired Life* (Random House, 2025), xviii.
14. David Whyte, "Seeking Language Large Enough," interview by Krista Tippett, *On Being*, April 7, 2016, https://onbeing.org/programs/david-whyte-seeking-language-large-enough/.
15. Megan Devine, *It's OK That You're Not OK: Meeting Grief and Loss in a Culture That Doesn't Understand* (Sounds True, 2017), 151.
16. Parker Palmer, "A Great People to Be Gathered: The View from Pendle Hill," *Friends Journal*, June 1, 2011, https://www.friendsjournal.org/great-people-be-gathered-view-pendle-hill/.
17. Parker Palmer, *Let Your Life Speak: Listening to the Voice of Vocation* (Jossey-Bass, 1999).
18. Toko-Pa Turner, "Clearing the Fog," May 7, 2020, https://toko-pa.com/2020/05/07/clearing-the-fog/.
19. Rev. angel Kyodo williams, "Love as Spaciousness," interview by Krista Tippett, *On Being*, April 7, 2016, https://onbeing.org/programs/rev-angel-kyodo-williams-on-love-as-spaciousness/.

20. Melissa Febos, “Ode to an Outcast Part,” in *The Book of Alchemy: A Creative Practice for an Inspired Life*, Suleika Jaouad, author (Random House, 2025), 170.
21. Natalie Goldberg, “What Is the Way of Haiku?” *Creativity Portal* (blog), April 1, 2021, updated June 17, 2025, https://www.creativity-portal.com/articles/natalie-goldberg/three-simple-lines/the-way-haiku.html.
22. Tove Jansson, *The Summer Book* (Pantheon Books, 1974), 8.

INDEX

C

G

H

I

J

K

L

Y

ACKNOWLEDGMENTS

Before I settle into a book, I confess I read the acknowledgments first. I want to know about the soil from which it sprang, who the helpers were. So let me spoil the surprise here and say: legions. Legions of generous, giant souls have shepherded this book across years. Teachers, students, and clients who showed me what healing can look like. Friends, editors, and guides who grew this germ of an idea into the offering you now hold in your hands. And you, dear reader, the person I was writing toward, with the hope that something in here would ignite something in you, comfort or companionship or—my wildest hope—a way of loving yourself and your body into the world.

My deepest thanks to my wonderful agent Isabelle Bleecker, who believed in this project even when I utterly botched my pitch and then disappeared for a year, and who guided me with steady hand and tireless advocacy, offering wise expertise alongside a shared love of plants and gardening. Learning that the agency she and Jennifer Thompson spearhead was called Nordlyset, Norwegian for northern light, felt like an extra bit of Scandi kinship and kismet.

A huge bow of gratitude to my editor, Francesca Walker, whose generous and visionary guidance made this book infinitely more coherent and compelling. Our collaboration was a deep delight, as was working with the extraordinary folks at North Atlantic Books. Deep thanks to production editors Trisha Peck, Emily Boyd, and Gillian Hamel, copyeditor Adaobi Obi Tulton, and publicity director Julia Sadowski.

Thanks, too, to Molly Haley for photos, and for making even a radio face comfortable on camera.

To writer, teacher, and friend Susan Conley, without whom this book does not exist. When we met in a coffee shop a decade ago her unequivocal *YES, do this*, made me believe I could. She has revised, instructed, encouraged, immeasurably improved, and more than occasionally rescued my work.

Maine is lucky to have robust networks for writers and creative folks. Thank you to Hewnoaks Artist Residency, the Maine Arts Commission, and the Maine Writers and Publishers Association. To the organizations, schools, and centers that have offered wonderful spaces to teach and learn: the Monteverde Friends School, the Harvard Graduate School of Education, the Salt Institute for Documentary Studies, the Center for Documentary Studies at Duke University, the Public Radio Exchange (PRX.org), the Telling Room, Long Creek Youth Development Center, Blunt Youth Radio, In Her Presence, Good Medicine Collective, and the Biodynamic Craniosacral Association of North America.

Writing may be a solitary act, but my writer friends have shown me the opposite, nesting me in support, encouragement, and abiding generosity. Their own trailblazing works lit the path forward. Love and gratitude to Megan Devine, Matthew Burgess, Sarah Ramey, Deb Bicknell, Michael Erard, and Misty Mclaughlin, who somehow managed to companion me in daily writing from 6,000 miles away. Emily Bernhard for co-writing, Aja Evans for solidarity (and family!). Countless writing groups over the years offered spaces of generation and refinement, seeding pieces that landed here.

My wonderful, quirky origin family that wraps across the globe. To my ancestors and grandparents, and to my dad, David Franzel, and mom, Cecilia Franzel, each of whom—by example and design—helped me discover the truth of my own compass. My gratitude to them, and to their loving partners. To my sisters, Melina Dale and Julia Franzel, who buoy my soul and know laughter as medicine. A special *hejsan* to my Swedish family: Ingemar and Eivor Wetterholm, Magnus Wetterholm, Rune Jakobsson, Claes-Göran Wetterholm, and Bo Jerndell.

Gratitude for what's made living with chronic illness manageable, most especially Dr. Bridget Tremblay, Dr. Andreas Stefan, Kate Millbury, and Jason Stein: practitioners and doctors who show up with listening, expertise, and care. The land we live on has been oasis, nurturance, convalescence, and teacher. Wonderful neighbors who've built a community of care and mutual support. Enduring love to the animals, first Charlie and now Rosie, who demonstrate—every day, every breath—what it is to listen to your organism, to live truly, to rest deeply, to move in joy, and to pass on with grace.

Countless teachers have enriched my life and learning over years. An incomplete list includes deep indebtedness to Dr. Kate Klemer, Margaret Rosenau,

Lansing Barrett Gresham, Eric Davis, Steve Seidel, Jenny Rowe, Dot Fisher-Smith, John Barth, Rob Rosenthal, and Renie Allen.

To the wonderful contributors in these pages: Arly Scully, Susan Lebel Young, Marcella, Bridgett Brunea, Tessa Greene O'Brien, and Erika Arthur.

I've had the great honor of working with many clients and workshop participants who've generously shared their sorrows and celebrations, imbuing our embodied writing groups and sessions with intimacy, discovery, and connection. I'm deeply grateful to every single one of them and unendingly moved by their wholehearted practice of reverence and permission. Thanks also to *Permission Slips* Substack and newsletter readers whose encouragement and engagement over years have created deep conversations, even from afar.

A richness of beloveds: Sister Rosie: Colleen Kinsella and Molly Angie. Sage Hayes, Sarah Lawrie, Stacy Brenner, Kate Bathras and Tim Bathras (in memoriam), Lara Schneider, David Meiklejohn, Deb Gunther and Bill Tierney (in memoriam), Megan Poe, Bri Gallo (and letting go of the familiar), Alexa Williamson, Pilar Gizzi, Kate Cox, Matt Schreiber, Laura (Nerdy) Starecheski, and Megan Reed. Paul Sturtz and Polina Malikin, who blew on the embers of this book when they were nearly out, reanimating the whole thing (and connected me to Matthew Sharpe—thank you!). Our sister families: Chris and Kim Teret and Molly Angie and Chriss Sutherland, and the many children: Charlie, Suzanna, Javi, Kaya, and Phoenix.

And finally, where my heart lives outside my body: Meredith Crandall Brown, beloved sister BFF, and Sepideh Bajracharya, heart of my heart, soul twin. To Nora, Eagle Girl, whose incandescent creativity illuminates the way for us all, and whose wild intelligence, wry humor, and giant heart light my life and expand the possible. And to my love, Jon: punk rock Boy Scout, the best thing about America, forever first reader, who shows me that reverent depth and irreverent hilarity are not different places, and that worlds can be built through devoted care.

ABOUT THE AUTHOR

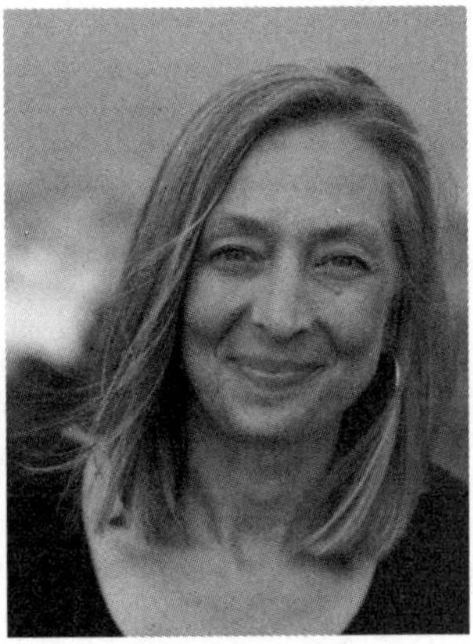

Photo by Molly Haley

Johanna Franzel is a writer, teacher, radio producer, and biodynamic craniosacral therapist who holds a master of arts in education from Harvard. She was the director of Generation PRX, a national network for youth radio stories for the Public Radio Exchange (PRX.org). After a chronic illness diagnosis in 2003, she drew on her expertise to develop embodied writing practices that became essential to reclaiming a new narrative of health. She's become a passionate advocate for sharing these practices, offering acclaimed workshops and writing to help others connect to their inner wisdom and vitality through language. She lives with her family outside Portland, Maine. Visit her at johannafranzel.com.

ABOUT NORTH ATLANTIC BOOKS

North Atlantic Books (NAB) is an independent, nonprofit publisher committed to a bold exploration of the relationships between mind, body, spirit, and nature. Founded in 1974, NAB aims to nurture a holistic view of the arts, sciences, humanities, and healing. To make a donation or to learn more about our books, authors, events, and newsletter, please visit www.northatlanticbooks.com.